HEMORRHOIDS

A Cure and Preventive

HEMORRHOIDS

A Cure and Preventive

by
Robert Lawrence Holt

Foreword and Addendum
by
Sanford Savin, M.D.

William Morrow and Company, Inc.
New York 1980

To the silent sufferers

First published by California Health Publications, 1977

Library of Congress Cataloging in Publication Data

Holt, Robert Lawrence.
Hemorrhoids.

Includes bibliographical references and index.
1. Hemorrhoids. 2. Cryosurgery. I. Title.
RC865.H64 1980 616.3′5 79-21792
ISBN 0-688-03584-1
ISBN 0-688-08584-9 pbk.

Printed in the United States of America.

First Morrow Edition

1 2 3 4 5 6 7 8 9 10

Illustrations by Gail Spratt

Book Design by Michael Mauceri

Foreword

The rectal torment of the author, Robert Holt, which was diagnosed as hemorrhoids, has resulted in an outstanding book on the subject. Though designed to educate the lay person, it will also benefit anyone in the health field, including physicians. The latest medical text books on hemorrhoids were published in the 1930's.

When Mr. Holt sought medical help for his distress, he became aware of the paucity of information on this common and disabling malady. He soon learned that there were many fellow sufferers and that none of them had any kind words about the conventional cutting hemorrhoidectomy performed in the hospital setting. He decided he would rather suffer than go through the torment of the cure and thus began his search.

In a circuitous manner, he learned that there was a technique of eliminating hemorrhoids by a freezing process called cryosurgery and, more precisely, cryohemorrhoidectomy. Again, when he went to his medical practitioners, they were unaware of the technique or who was able to perform it. He further investigated and eventually found the relief he sought, was cured of his distress by cryohemorrhoidectomy, and is now a staunch advocate and supporter of this form of treatment.

Robert Holt has compiled an immense fund of information on the subject of hemorrhoids including their cause, prevention, and modern-day treatment. None of his material is conjecture and it is all documented by exhaustive investigation of current medical literature and current medical research.

Although opinions expressed in the book, on occasion, may not necessarily be my own, I would concur in the majority of the conclusions drawn within the chapters of the book.

In closing, I should like to state that I first began performing cryogenic rectal surgery including cryohemorrhoidectomy in 1973 and now state without equivocation that it is not only an alternative to excisional hemorrhoidectomy but is by far the treatment of choice.

—Sanford Savin, M.D.

Chief of Proctology
Park City Hospital
Bridgeport, Connecticut

2660 Main St.
Bridgeport, Conn. 06606

Preface and Acknowledgments

A question which puzzled me more than any other during the writing of this book is "Why has there been no serious book written on the subject of hemorrhoids for the lay person?" There are literally thousands of books written for the lay person discussing ailments less prevalent than hemorrhoids. Why then are there not a great number of books already available on the subject of hemorrhoids? The most plausible, though not necessarily conclusive, answer to this question may be that as long as excisional hemorrhoidectomy (surgery) was the primary solution offered by modern medicine, we sufferers really didn't care to know much more about the problem—there was no acceptable solution for us. It was an embarrassing problem which we seldom discussed with our peers; and the medical solutions we knew of we abhorred. So, it is little wonder that no one has seriously written on this subject before.

The reason that I have written this book is to tell the millions of hemorrhoid sufferers that there is a solution now which is *acceptable*. Modern medicine has finally developed and refined a technique in which discomfort is minimized and the patient can expect to resume a normal work routine quickly.

As with any new medical technique, a great deal of time can transpire before the medical community studies, tests, and eventually begins to generally apply such a procedure.

During this interim period, it can be very difficult for a lay person to find a source of such treatment. I am much indebted to several individuals who provided both guiding knowledge and encouragement to pursue this subject. In particular, Barry Kramer (staff reporter for *The Wall Street Journal*), Patrick Kelley (representative of Ritter Company), and Dr. James Patrick Fleming of Rochester, New York, should be mentioned.

Introducing new medical techniques in any field of medicine can be a trying affair, requiring both courage and fortitude.

The physician best known for developing and introducing the technique of cryosurgery in treating hemorrhoids is Dr. Martin I. Lewis, of Irvine, California.

A number of other prominent surgeons in North America and England have refined Dr. Lewis' technique to its current state. Their work has been published in the medical journals of their respective countries. They are:

James Barron	Boca Raton, Fla.
J. J. Bernhard	Phoenix, Ariz.
Salvatore J. Detrano	Christ Hospital, Jersey City, N.J.
Howard J. Eddy	Veteran's Hospital, Northport, N.Y.
James P. Fleming	Rochester, N.Y.
J. C. Goligher	Univ. Dept. of Surgery, Leeds, England
H. D. Kaufman	Selly Oak Hospital, Birmingham, England
William Leebron	Elk City, Okla.
Bert Myers	Univ. of New Orleans, La.
John J. O'Connor	Georgetown Univ., Washington, D.C.
Changyul Oh	Mt. Sinai School of Medicine, New York
William W. H. Rudd	Toronto, Canada
Sanford Savin	Bridgeport, Conn.
Philip F. Schofield	Park Hospital, Manchester, England
Stanley P. Wegryn	Sanibel Island, Fla.
K. Lloyd Williams	St. Martin's Hospital, Somerset, England
Martin Wilson	Park Hospital, Manchester, England

When the answer to the question "What is a hemorrhoid?" is finally agreed upon by the medical community, we will probably have the following physicians and researchers to thank for defining this difficult and widely misunderstood subject:

Denis P. Burkitt	Medical Research Council, London
Mandel Ganchrow	Spring Valley, N.Y.
C. W. Graham-Stewart	Harrogate General Hospital, England
Peter H. Lord	London, England
Neil S. Painter	Manor House Hospital, London
J. P. Partridge	Barnstaple, England
A. F. Pineda	Nat. Univ. of La Plata, Argentina
G. C. Prasad	Banaras Hindu University, India
R. E. B. Tagart	Newmarket Gen. Hospital, England
Hamish Thomson	Gloucestershire Royal Hosp., England
Hugh C. Trowell	Fordingbridge, England
William S. Slack	Middlesex Hospital, England

A very special note of gratitude is given to the unknown public servant at the Federal Trade Commission who generously (and anonymously) photocopied and mailed to me the 124 pages of the "Complaint, Initial Decision, Opinion, Findings, Conclusions, and Final Order (August 28, 1964–December 16, 1966)," which related the "usefulness" of one of the most popular commercial preparations for hemorrhoids.

The author is indebted to the staff of Senator Alan Cranston for providing the research sources which explain why the above "Final Order" of the FTC was later modified in 1969 and 1970. It is clearly evident that general confusion and ignorance surrounding the widely misunderstood subjects of hemorrhoids and anal blood clots (a complication thereof) extends to members of the Federal Trade Commission and U.S. Court of Appeals also.

Of great value to me has been the professional assistance rendered by Dr. Sanford Savin, the Chief of Proctology at Park City Hospital in Bridgeport, Connecticut. Few, if any, physicians have done more to refine the initial cryosurgical technique introduced by Dr. Martin I. Lewis in 1969. The readers of this book are especially fortunate that Dr. Savin agreed to permit an article by him on cryosurgery to be included as an addendum to this book.

I hope that this book may lead to considerably more research as to the nature of hemorrhoids and their proper treatment, in addition to a higher level of governmental and corporate responsibility in the marketing of commercial products sold to the millions of hemorrhoid sufferers.

—R.L.H.

Contents

List of Illustrations

PART I

The Problem

Chapter 1

Introduction

This is a patient-oriented book. It should provide the reader with a clear and complete understanding of the nature, causes, symptoms, and proper treatment of hemorrhoids. Confusion and misconceptions concerning this subject exist not only among the public, but also within the medical profession.

Having suffered over a decade from this condition and then having found a relatively painless cure, I hope my experiences will provide valuable insight as to how you too may free yourself of this problem.

INCIDENCE

From the sparse information on hemorrhoids to be found in popular magazines and the few people who openly complain of them, we might assume that hemorrhoids are a rare occurrence. Quite the contrary, they are considered by many medical authorities to be one of the most common persisting, serious, physical ailments occurring in Western industrialized societies.[1,2,3]

In the United States, *Time* magazine has referred to hemorrhoids as:

> just about the commonest complaint seen by the surgeon . . . one of the least-talked about but most advertised of human conditions.[4]

In a medical study at the world-famous Mayo Clinic, it was found that more than half (52 percent) of those examined proctoscopically had hemorrhoids.[5] Proctoscopy is an examination of the anal canal and rectum utilizing a short telescopic instrument.

The medical textbook *Diseases of the Colon and Anorectum* (Turrell, Vol. II, 1959) discloses that:

> most people develop hemorrhoids of some degree beginning about the age of 20, which become progressively larger during their physically active life.[6]

Although most individuals may begin to develop hemorrhoids in their twenties, the hemorrhoidal symptoms usually do not become evident until the thirties. In a review of the records of 23,446 patients with hemorrhoids, it was found that 80 percent of the patients were between the ages of thirty and sixty. Eight percent were less than thirty years of age.[7]

On October 14, 1976, at the annual Clinical Congress of the American College of Surgeons, Dr. Matthew A. Larkin (chairman of surgery at Mercy Hospital in Miami, Florida) stated that "all people have hemorrhoids by the time they are in their seventies." [8]

In *The Wall Street Journal* (August 10, 1973) we are told:

> experts believe that among humans there are more adults with hemorrhoids than without them.

This same article suggests that as many as *forty million* adult Americans have symptomatic hemorrhoids.

Perhaps the most precise statement was made at a symposium, "Diverse Methods of Managing Hemorrhoids," held during the annual meeting of the American Proctologic Society in New York City from June 11 to 14, 1972. At this symposium, Dr. James A. Ferguson of Grand Rapids, Michigan, stated.

> one hundred percent of the population has hemorrhoids and fifty percent of them may be symptomatic.[9]

It may be surprising to learn that more than half of our adult acquaintances have developed some degree of hemorrhoids with noticeable symptoms.

THE SILENT SUFFERER

Persons who are victims of hemorrhoids are usually very hesitant to discuss their problem. It is a subject concerning an area of the body which many people would prefer not discussing, especially if it is a problem area.

How often have you heard the subject discussed in a living room among company, at a cocktail party, among coworkers at your job, or even between close friends and relatives? The subject is not exactly "table conversation."

It was not until months after my hemorrhoids were treated that I was willing to discuss the matter openly with persons other than my immediate family. I was surprised to learn that a brother and one of my parents suffered from hemorrhoids. Later, I learned that four of my closest business associates also had the problem.

During the preparation of this book, I have encouraged others to discuss their hemorrhoidal problems. Many people find it very difficult to do so. Having been there myself, I can understand and sympathize.

HISTORY OF HEMORRHOIDS

Hemorrhoids have been medically treated for many thousands of years. In Ancient Egypt the practice of proctology as a specialty flourished.[10] The ailment was known in the time of Hippocrates, whose writings contain references to various treatments for hemorrhoids, including *excision* (surgery) and *ligation* (binding).[11] Until the last decade the medical profession could offer little more than the same treatments which were available more than two thousand years ago.

For a long time it was generally believed, due to symptomatic bleeding, that the presence of hemorrhoids was beneficial to the human body.[12] This was at a time when many physicians drew blood from their patients, believing such an act would help restore health. The English word, hemorrhoid, is derived from the Greek *haimorrhoides* meaning blood flow.[13] The Italian version, *profluvio di sangue*, means overflow of blood.[14]

Until this century, hemorrhoids were considered an affliction of the wealthier classes [15]; at one time, almost the exclusive illness of the nobility and royalty. This may help explain the derivation of the French and German words for hemorrhoid:

> French—*flux d'or* or flow of gold;
> German—*goldene Ader* or golden veins.[16]

One of the most famous battles in history, the Battle of Waterloo, may have been determined by the debilitating effects of hemorrhoids on the Emperor Napoleon. The medical historian Rudolph Marx has written:

> Napoleon's painful piles, which he has had since his youth, were so inflamed and excruciating, and the emperor was so groggy from lack of sleep and from the opium given him to relieve his suffering, that he couldn't get out of bed, let alone sit on his horse.[17]

Those of us who have suffered the agony of an anal blood clot (a symptom of hemorrhoids) can appreciate what Napoleon's problem must have been. Historical records indicate that Napoleon's diet while he ruled France may have contributed greatly to his problem.[18] The subject of diet as a cause of hemorrhoids receives attention later (in Chapter 5).

Occasionally, the word "piles" is also used to describe the condition of hemorrhoids. This word is derived from the Latin *pila,* which means a ball or swelling.[19] Although this word is a more accurate description of the condition, it is seldom found in references or general conversation.

LIMITED INFORMATION

A problem which has confronted all hemorrhoid sufferers is a dismaying lack of information concerning the subject. According to the periodical guides found in our public libraries (up to mid-1977), there have been only four articles in popular magazines devoted to the subject in the last ten years. These include one column each in *Newsweek* and *Time* magazine and two brief articles in *McCall's*[20] and *Vogue.*[21] If you read few women's magazines and missed the January 13, 1967, issue of *Time* and the November 1, 1976, issue of *Newsweek,* then you may have had little opportunity to read anything concerning your affliction.

On August 10, 1973, an article on hemorrhoids appeared in the widely distributed financial newspaper, *The Wall Street Journal.* This article, written by Barry Kramer, was quite informative. Its comprehensiveness is indicated by the title and subtitle:

> Medical Advances, Some New Cures Help Hemorrhoid Sufferers, Whose Number Is Legion. Among Methods: Freezing; Debunking Some Myths

This was the first article in any publication that I had read on the subject. It offered considerable hope to individuals such as myself who were unwilling to undergo surgery to solve their problem.

To the best of my knowledge, Mr. Kramer's article was also the first time that *freezing* was mentioned as a treatment for hemorrhoids in any widely read publication in the United States. This procedure is called *cryosurgery* (also referred to as cryotherapy, cryohemorrhoidectomy, cryotechnique, or cryodestruction in various references). The emphasis of this article is that cryosurgery offers the patient comparatively little discomfort and fewer complications than a traditional hemorrhoidectomy. The article opened the door to eventual curative treatment for me, as I'm sure it has for countless others who were fortunate to have read the article.

SOURCES OF MISINFORMATION

Shortly after this article appeared in *The Wall Street Journal,* I was treated by a proctologist (a physician specializing in illnesses of the anorectum) for my second blood clot. A blood clot is a by-product and symptom of hemorrhoids. I asked this physician what was the cause of my hemorrhoids? Also, what preventative measures, including dietary, could I take? He told me that straining was probably the primary cause of hemorrhoids, but that he knew of no way to prevent their occurrence by altering the diet. As this book will clearly reveal and document, it is poor dietary intake that results in constipation, which in turn causes the straining that the physician correctly named as the cause of my hemorrhoids.

The same physician told me that the only solution to my problem was the surgical removal of my hemorrhoids. This was five years after cryotherapy had been developed as a curative treatment and several thousand years after ligation (binding) had been developed as an alternative to surgery.[22] When I asked the physician for his opinion of cryotherapy, he told me that such a procedure could lead to scar formation, which in turn might affect one's control of the anal canal. This sounded like a rather strong indictment of the new procedure, and as my problem was not yet severe, I mistakenly decided to postpone any curative treatment at that time. It was much later (three years) that I learned that one of the many advantages of cryotherapy is that it very rarely leaves scar tissue.[23,24] In fact, it is the technique of *surgical* removal that can result in the formation of scar tissue.[25]

Other sources of misinformation are the advertising claims

and other information provided by the manufacturers of commercial hemorrhoidal suppositories. This advertising is frequently directed at a complication of hemorrhoids—the anal blood clot. The nature, progress, and medical treatment of anal blood clots differ considerably from those of hemorrhoids.

According to the editors of *Consumer Reports,* "there is no acceptable evidence substantiating advertised claims that Preparation H can shrink hemorrhoids, reduce inflammation, and heal injured tissue." [26]

An official publication of the American Pharmaceutical Association states that the use of these self-medications due to "unsupported advertising claims" can "have serious consequences" in that the patient may fail to seek proper medical advice.[27] As with many medical problems, the longer they are ignored, the more serious they will become.[28]

These same manufacturers suggest the use of laxatives to hemorrhoid sufferers (see their product instructions). As we shall see later in this book, the frequent use of laxatives is believed to be one of the main causes of constipation,[29] which, in turn, is the chief cause of hemorrhoids.

Perhaps the worst advice these manufacturers can provide to persons with hemorrhoids is to suggest the consumption of a low-residue (fiber) diet, yet this advice is found in the instructions enclosed in the boxes of suppositories sold by a major drug manufacturer. This is the very diet that the majority of medical opinion in the Western world now believes is the most responsible for constipation and consequent straining.[30,31,32,33,34,35]

IDENTIFYING THE PROBLEM

There is some difficulty in treating a condition such as hemorrhoids that has so many conflicting definitions. The problems involved in clarifying this medical subject are well stated by Dr. Leon Banov, Jr., of Charleston, South Carolina:

> This generation has inherited the word "hemorrhoid"

> along with a large variety of definitions of hemorrhoids. . . . And when you discover confusion within the medical profession, you will have understandable pity for the lay person who regards nearly all anorectal ailments as hemorrhoids.[36]

The five chapters immediately following are devoted to defining the nature of the anal canal and how hemorrhoids develop within this passage. Since there is a confusing plethora of definitions available, this book will generally use the terminology of modern *British* medical practice (the term "cryotherapy" is used instead of "cryosurgery").

We must look also to British medicine for research into the causes of hemorrhoids. That we must look abroad for such research is probably due to the greater effort in England in the field of preventive medicine. This emphasis seems to be prevalent in many nations which offer free medical care to their citizens.

The state of research in the United States in the area of preventive medicine is summarized by Harold J. Taub, executive director of *Prevention* magazine in the following:

> Most American medical journals won't publish anything unless it is already well-accepted by the medical profession, so nobody ever learns anything new by reading them. When a doctor has something new and important to report, he usually does it in England.[37]

From this research, one of our first "discoveries" is that hemorrhoids are not veins. It has been determined that a hemorrhoid is part of an *arteriovenal cushion*, of which there are three within the anal canal.[38] The *arteriovenal connections* within these cushions consist of arteries and veins which are directly connected, with no intervening capillaries.[39] This helps to explain why hemorrhoidal bleeding is always bright red.[40,41] This, of course, is not a characteristic of the blood that flows in the veins. Therefore, the common opinion that hemorrhoids are varicose veins of the rectum is false.[42,43]

The fact that an anal blood clot is not a hemorrhoid has

already been discussed. The two conditions differ in many important respects, particularly in their symptoms, progress, and medical treatment.[44] Since a blood clot is accompanied by considerably more pain and discomfort than hemorrhoids, and at times may require immediate medical attention, a separate chapter has been included on this subject (Chapter 4).

THE FIRST SYMPTOMS

In addition to a blood clot, other symptoms which may suggest the existence of hemorrhoids are: bleeding and a small, protruding lump of tissue at the anal opening. All of these symptoms may become evident during or after a bowel movement. Medical opinion differs as to which symptom will be noticed first. Which is noticed first is not as important as what you do when you notice it.

When your first symptom occurs, there are a number of measures that should be *immediately* undertaken. The most important, especially if the first sign is bleeding, is to arrange for a proper examination by a qualified physician, preferably a proctologist. In the majority of instances, the bleeding is probably due to the passage of hard fecal matter, complicated by the presence of a few hemorrhoids.[45] This is possible even if the hemorrhoids do not yet protrude at the conclusion of a bowel movement. An examination can easily confirm the presence of the hemorrhoids, or any of a number of other potential problems. When your first symptom is a blood clot, the physician may conduct only a digital examination if the swelling of the clot is substantial. A digital examination is the use of a finger to investigate the condition of the anal canal and the outer portion of the rectum.

It is normal to have some hesitation or embarrassment about this examination. Such hesitation to seek medical attention is no longer well founded. Within the last few years, a number of new methods of detecting serious anorectal and intestinal disorders have been developed. These methods do not necessarily involve the somewhat uncomfortable physical examinations of the past. These new techniques are thoroughly discussed in the chapter on examinations (Chapter 16).

A few medical references suggest that patients with a hemorrhoidal symptom are sometimes hesitant to see a physician for fear that they have a more serious disorder. I have shared this fear, but this is not a good reason to postpone positive action. All of the other disorders can be successfully treated in their early stages, often by such conservative treatment as a change in diet.[46]

PERSONAL TREATMENT

After making an appointment for an examination, you should give some thought to your recent intake of food and drink. If it has resulted in constipation, you may have a good idea of what not to consume in the future. For a detailed description of the preferred foods and drinks to alleviate constipation and prevent the problem, Chapters 7 and 8 should be helpful.

By improving your diet while your hemorrhoids are in an early stage, you may be able to arrest further development, and in fact cause the anal canal to return to normal.[47]

A number of individuals will find it necessary to adjust personal habits other than diet in order to improve their condition. Once a person has developed the habit of straining during defecation, altering this habit may become just as important as modifying the diet. I have a close relative whose master bathroom contains a good-sized television set. This same relative has hemorrhoids of an advanced degree. Correct bathroom procedure is outlined in Chapter 9.

After reading the initial chapters of this book, the reader may realize just how important the overall health of the body is to the prevention of hemorrhoids. Although the relationship may seem remote, proper exercise is vital to the smooth functioning of the cushions within the anal canal.[48] If you follow all the other suggestions in this book in order to prevent the further development of your hemorrhoids, the lack of proper exercise alone may preclude your success. Many references to this effect will be found in the following pages.

If your hemorrhoids are firmly established by this time (as mine were), your first priority will be to seek prompt medical attention. By "firmly established" is meant that the hemorrhoids protrude at the conclusion of a bowel movement, requiring manual replacement. In addition, slight bleeding may frequently be noticed during the passage of hard stools or when the hemorrhoids are abraded during replacement.

The particular proctologist with whom you make an appointment is all-important in determining which medical techniques will be available to cure your problem. New advances in the field of medicine can take many, many years to gain popular practice. Should you make an appointment with a proctologist who still practices traditional hemorrhoidectomy (excisional surgery), you should know what to expect.

TRADITIONAL MEDICAL TREATMENT

This method of "corrective surgery is infamous for its pain and complications." These are the words of Dr. Salvatore J. Detrano, the director of proctology at Christ Hospital in Jersey City, New Jersey.[49]

In the words of another physician, Dr. R. E. B. Tagart of Suffolk, England, it is one of:

> the methods that has gained the unenviable and counterproductive reputation of being more painful than the condition they aim to alleviate.[50]

It is little wonder that less than one percent of all Americans thought to have hemorrhoids submit to this form of treatment each year.[51] The "myriad" complications following traditional hemorrhoidectomy, especially pain, help to explain why so few doctors who suffer from hemorrhoids are willing to undergo surgical hemorrhoidectomy.[52]

Patients who submit to this form of treatment can expect:

1. a general or spinal anesthetic,

2. three to ten days of hospitalization, and
3. a home recovery of one to four weeks.[11]

Postoperative complications may include:

1. excruciating pain, requiring pain-killing drugs,
2. urinary retention (inability to urinate), requiring catheterization,
3. heavy bleeding,
4. stricture (narrowing of the anal canal),
5. fissure formation (cleft or crack in the lining of the anal canal), and
6. scar formation.[54,55,56,57]

Notwithstanding the above conditions and complications, traditional hemorrhoidectomy has been one of the most frequently performed operations in the hospitals of the United States.[58] In 1973 *The Wall Street Journal* reported that "an estimated 400,000 hemorrhoidectomies . . . are performed annually."[59]

Perhaps the impressions of a nurse who has had considerable experience assisting hemorrhoidectomy patients during their postoperative period can best describe the ordeal:

> I discovered that strong men who had known severe hardship, or had suffered serious wounds during the war, could be reduced to shamed, pain-ridden humiliation after an operation for piles.
>
> I would have preferred to face hordes of bayonet-waving enemy soldiers than to have to give that first crucificial olive-oil enema to an already demoralised man.
>
> Later, in the female ward, women patients swore that their worst labor pains were mild compared with the throbbing pains of piles or piles removed.[60]

Fortunately, this method of excisional surgery is being rapidly replaced by a number of other forms of medical treatment which do not have all the disadvantages that deter the patient from seeking medical relief.

NEW METHODS OF TREATMENT

Recently, it was announced that the number of people requiring surgery for their hemorrhoids over the past fifteen years has been reduced by 75 percent, due to the development of other effective treatments. This was announced at a news conference on October 14, 1976, at the conclusion of the annual Clinical Congress of the American College of Surgeons in Chicago.[61]

These new techniques are injection, ligation, and cryosurgery. The injection method has been practiced for a number of years and is used primarily for the elderly and other patients who might not tolerate other forms of medical treatment. This method is not suggested for others, since the hemorrhoids "generally return in three to five years," according to Dr. Eugene P. Salvati, chief of surgery at Muhlenberg Hospital in Plainfield, New Jersey.[62]

Ligation involves the binding of the hemorrhoids by the use of small rubber rings. Recent adaptations of this ancient remedy have greatly improved its effectiveness and acceptance by patients. This method is more effective than injection since the hemorrhoids recur in only five percent of the cases.[63] Depending on the size and location of the hemorrhoid, this method may be accompanied by some degree of discomfort. An infrequent complication of ligation is the formation of blood clots near the treated tissue and postoperative hemorrhage.[64,65,66]

The patient may also be required to return to the physician's office several times, as only one hemorrhoid should be treated per session.[67]

The use of cryosurgery, a freezing of the hemorrhoidal tissue, overcomes most of the initial disadvantages of excision, injection and ligation and greatly lessens the complications which may occur later.

CRYOSURGERY

The use of cryogenics, a branch of physics that relates to the production and effects of very low temperatures, in the field of medicine dates back to the turn of the century. Its initial use was in dermatology, as early as 1898.[68] At that time, low temperatures were obtained through the use of carbon dioxide. It was not until 1950, when liquid nitrogen was introduced, that the full potential of cryogenics in medicine began to be realized. Cryosurgery is now used extensively in neurosurgery, gynecology, ophthalmology, urology, ear-nose-and-throat surgery, and rectal surgery. In the field of rectal surgery, success has been reported in using this technique in the treatment of fissures, fistulas, anal polyps, condylomata, and hemorrhoids.

The procedure of cryosurgery involves delivering a freezing temperature to the hemorrhoidal tissue. The hemorrhoid is thereby frozen, destroying the cells of the tissue. The technique requires only a few minutes per hemorrhoid and can be performed in a physician's office as well as in hospital facilities.

After the procedure the patient can expect to return to a normal work routine within a few days.[69] Self-employed individuals often return to work sooner than others, frequently the day following treatment (as I did).[70]

Some discomfort can be expected as the freezing temperature is applied to the hemorrhoid. Most physicians apply a desensitizing agent or inject a local anesthetic in the area of the anal canal before treatment. With some techniques, the use of an anesthetic is optional, depending on the preference of the patient.

Direct Freezing

Both internal and external hemorrhoidal tissue can be directly frozen, either in a one-stage treatment or multiple sessions.

The delivery of the freezing temperature to the hemorrhoidal tissue initially causes this tissue to swell. Direct freezing of hemorrhoids may result in a water discharge from the swollen tissue for a number of days, requiring the patient to use an absorbent pad.[71] The drainage from hemorrhoids frozen internally may be slight, while drainage from hemorrhoids frozen externally may be considerable.

Ligation Before Freezing

The ligation of hemorrhoidal tissue prior to freezing is limited to that tissue which lies beneath the mucosal lining of the anal canal.[72] Such ligation precludes the normal circulation of blood in the tissue during the freezing, and some physicians feel that this provides for a better freezing of the tissue.

In both techniques, the treated hemorrhoidal tissue sloughs away from the lining of the anal canal a week to two weeks later. The degree of discomfort experienced during this post-operative period varies, but most physicians report that less than ten percent of their patients require analgesics (pain-killers).[73]

The concluding chapters of the book discuss how to find a cryosurgeon, the examination procedure, and the various techniques of cryosurgery. The information concerning these subjects has been extracted from the research reports and letters of eighteen physicians who have been leaders in developing and refining this new method of treating hemorrhoids. They report on their successful treatment of more than four thousand patients in the United States and England.

I hope the following information will provide you with both the incentive and confidence to seek proper care for your problem.

Chapter 2

The Internal Sphincter

The internal sphincter of the anal canal is designed to regulate the frequency of bowel movements. The functioning of the internal sphincter is the key to understanding the development of hemorrhoids.

This control mechanism is quite simple—the internal sphincter will naturally open when it is dilated by a bowel movement of adequate size and sufficient bulk (consistency).

The cervix of a woman in labor functions in a similar fashion. Before the baby can naturally exit from the mother's womb, the cervix must be dilated to a width of ten centimeters. The reflex to push will not occur until this dilation is completed.

OUR ELIMINATION SYSTEM

The internal sphincter is an important component of a complicated elimination system—our anal canal and rectum.

The scarcity of information concerning this general subject may account for some of the difficulty in finding accurate information concerning the related subject of hemorrhoids. Anatomical descriptions of this portion of the human body are rarely found in ordinary references.

It is necessary to review how the human elimination system works in order to better understand how a hemorrhoid develops. The following description assumes that a proper diet is being consumed, thereby permitting the body to function naturally.

The Anal Canal

The anal canal is an intricate system of sphincters, blood vessels, cavities within these blood vessels, connective elastic tissue and muscle fiber, nerves, and other body tissue.

The length of the canal is one-and-one-quarter inches.

THE ANAL CANAL

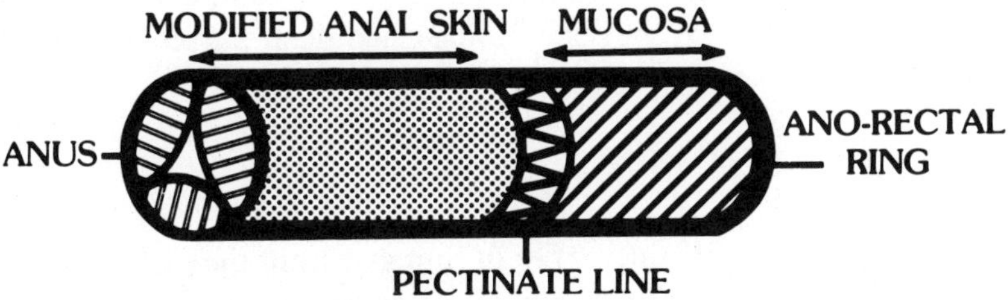

The Anal Sphincters

A sphincter is a ring-shaped muscle that controls the opening of a body passage. The anal canal has two sphincters.

The external sphincter (anus) controls the exit of the anal canal. This sphincter is consciously controlled by the individual, and therefore is referred to as a *voluntary* muscle.

The internal sphincter controls the entrance to the anal canal from the rectum. This sphincter is not consciously controlled, and therefore is considered an *involuntary* muscle. As mentioned earlier, two conditions within the rectum are required to cause the natural opening of this sphincter:

1. fullness of the rectum, and
2. relative firmness of the stool (a moist, bulky consistency).[1,2]

The reason for these particular requirements is that the body must have some means of controlling the required frequency of bowel movements. Without this regulatory mechanism, it might be necessary to have bowel movements as often as feces are delivered into the rectum by peristalsis—which can be three to four times daily. By requiring bulky stools that fill the rectum to initiate a bowel movement, the internal sphincter is an invaluable body mechanism.

Anorectal Ring

The junction of the anal canal and the rectum is surrounded by a boundary called the anorectal ring. This boundary is well defined, as the anal mucosa (lining) is a deep purple and the rectal mucosa has a pinkish hue.

Linings of the Canal

There are two distinct types of linings within the anal canal. They are separated by a boundary called the *pectinate line* (also referred to as the "dentate line" or "line of anal valves"). This line has a serrated appearance and is located approximately three-quarters of an inch inside the canal.

The Anal Skin. The outer two-thirds of the canal is lined with a modified anal skin. This skin has neither the hair nor the sweat glands of ordinary skin. It is as sensitive as ordinary skin, though, a fact that is quite apparent when a blood clot forms beneath it.

The Mucosa. The inner third of the canal is lined with a mucous membrane, or mucosa. This membrane is far less sensitive than the modified anal skin. A blood clot located beneath the mucosa may pass unnoticed unless complications occur.[3]

The mucosa is sensitive to stretching. This sensitivity must be considered by the physician during an examination, as the components of the lower intestinal tract tend to tighten when stretched.

The Anal Cushions

Beneath the linings of the anal canal is a network of blood vessels, both veins and arteries. This network is divided into three masses, or cushions. Each cushion extends the length of the anal canal. With the body viewed in a standing position, these cushions converge around the circle of the anus at three o'clock, seven o'clock, and eleven o'clock.

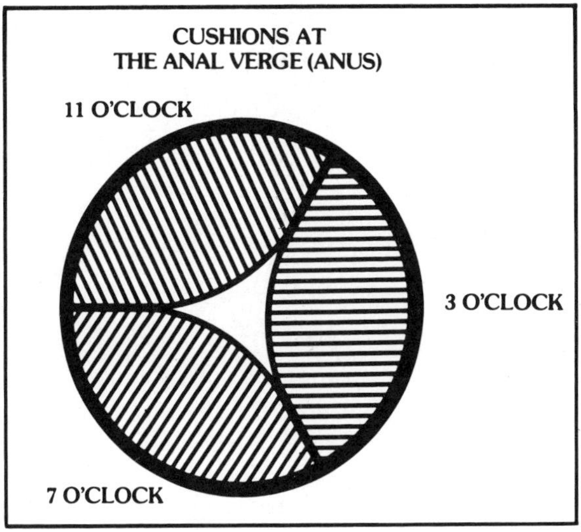

Arteriovenal Connections. Each of the cushions is connected to a branch of the superior rectal artery. The arteries in these cushions connect directly with the veins without intervening capillaries. This is an unusual arrangement, since capillaries normally form a bridge between the arteries and veins of the body.

Cavities. Instead of capillaries, the arteries and veins have connective spaces or cavities, also referred to as *nodules,* and *glomerules*. The presence of these cavities creates a cavernous body of tissue within the anal cushions.[4,5] In the absence of capillaries, blood can quickly enter and exit the area of the cushions. The cavernous structure also permits great changes in the size of the cushion complex.

Connective Elastic Tissue. A network of elastic tissue and smooth muscle fiber anchors the anal cushions to the internal sphincter of the anal canal.[6] These supportive tissues are designed to hold the cushions generally in place during bowel movements.

Function of the Anal Cushions

The unique tissue structure of the anal cushions enables the body to effectively close the interior of the anal canal between bowel movements.

Dr. A. F. Pineda, professor of anatomy at the National University in La Plata, Argentina, has observed that the arteries in the anal canal connect to a tissue structure:

> . . . similar to the spongy substance of the cavernous body of the genitals . . . the arriving blood acts as a filling which makes said formation ingurgitate, and together with the sphincter muscular system, is also an important element in the self-control of the rectum-anus.[7]

The findings of Dr. Pineda are confirmed by the research of Dr. Hamish Thomson, physician at Gloucestershire Royal Hospital, Gloucester, England.[8] As the stool passes through the anal canal, it displaces the blood in the cushions. Under normal, healthy conditions, the blood easily exits from the area of the three cushions during the bowel movements.

PROCESS OF ELIMINATION

There are four steps in the process of elimination. Peristalsis is the catalyst for this process. This reaction is the result of the stomach being filled with food. The fullness causes a wavelike, alternate contraction and dilation of the intestinal tract, which pushes the contents of the intestinal tract forward. These waves occur three to four times a day, usually following a meal.

Step One—Arrival of Feces at the Rectum

A direct result of peristalsis is the delivery of fecal matter into the pouch of the rectum. The amount of fecal matter delivered into the rectum is dependent upon three factors:

1. the amount of food consumed in daily meals,
2. the type of food consumed, and
3. the length of time which has elapsed since these meals.

The rectum should reach its maximum fullness approximately thirty-six hours after the consumption of the largest daily meal.[9] This is the length of time that the body requires to digest and eliminate a healthy diet.

Step Two—Contractions of the Rectum

The fullness of the stomach also initiates contractions of the rectum. This stimulates a desire for a bowel movement, a reaction especially evident in young children. As we approach adulthood, this desire is often suppressed by cultural factors and poor habits. Dr. Roy C. Darlington of the department of pharmacy at Howard University reveals the result of suppressing this natural urge:

> . . . if defecation is not allowed to occur when the defecation reflexes are excited, they become progressively less strong.[10]

When the urge for a bowel movement is suppressed over a lengthy period of time, the rectal nerves may lose their sensitivity and therefore their ability to assist in the natural functioning of the bowels.

Step Three—Dilation of the Internal Sphincter

When the stools are of sufficient size and consistency, they will naturally cause the dilation (opening) of the internal sphincter.[11] This makes the consumption of the proper foods a particularly important factor in correct bowel functioning.

Dr. Denis P. Burkitt, the well-known British surgeon, tells us:

> . . . defecation should be almost effortless, and the feces, which should be soft and bulky, are expelled by contractions of the gut and not by the muscles of the abdominal wall.[12]

Step Four—Relaxation of the External Sphincter

The last step in the process of elimination is the voluntary relaxation of the external anal sphincter. This permits the rectal muscles to expel the feces. As Dr. Burkitt says, this should be accomplished with little or no conscious effort.

After the bowel movement has begun, the length of time required for the expulsion of the feces should seldom exceed one minute.

The body's system for elimination is well designed and will function properly for a lifetime when due consideration is given to one's food intake. Difficulty in bowel functioning may be a measure of shortcomings in both personal diet and toilet habits.

Chapter 3

Hemorrhoids and Complications of Hemorrhoids

From the preceding chapter, we have learned that:

1. when engorged with blood, the three anal cushions act to close the interior of the anal canal.
2. the anal cushions are held in place by elastic connective tissue.
3 the anal canal's internal sphincter requires a large, bulky stool to be naturally dilated.
4. the act of emptying one's bowels should be accomplished with little or no conscious effort.

CONSTRICTION OF THE ANAL CANAL

The initial development of a hemorrhoid can be due to a number of varying factors. These variations are due to the individual dietary and toilet habits of each patient. These factors may work singly or in combination to encourage the development of hemorrhoids. The end result is a narrowing of the anal opening.

Inadequate Dilation of the Sphincters

It is normal for muscles of the body to constrict in size when they are not used. There is no reason why the anal sphincter muscles should be any different in this regard.

Dr. Peter H. Lord, a British surgeon with extensive experience in the nonsurgical treatment of hemorrhoids, has observed that hemorrhoid patients have a narrowed or constricted anal canal. He states:

> These pads (anal cushions) of vascular tissue normally give no trouble, but in patients who suffer from hemorrhoids there is a narrowing or constriction of the outlet so that during defecation the intrarectal pressure rises sufficiently to obstruct venous return from these vascular pads, which therefore become engorged. As these pads swell up, they further restrict the outlet.[1]

The reason for the improper dilation of the anal sphincters is the lack of consistently large and bulky stools. This, in turn, is due to dietary deficiencies, a subject to be discussed fully later in Chapter 8.

The lack of proper dilation of the sphincter muscles will eventually contribute to the narrowing of the anal canal.

Any constriction of the anal canal will necessitate additional straining during bowel movements. This straining over a prolonged period of time encourages the development of hemorrhoids.

Habitual Straining

All too often, bowel movements are accompanied by *habitual* straining, either to assist or to force the elimination of the feces.

Such straining prevents the natural exit of the stools because it results in reverse flow of blood in the veins which drain the anal canal and rectum.[2] This reverse flow of blood is harmful for two reasons:

1. it prevents or retards the escape of blood from the anal cushions as the stool passes through, and
2. it may also result in further engorgement within the anal cushions of blood from the veins.

The result of this straining is described by the British surgeon Dr. Tagart:

> The shearing force of a fecal bolus (stool) passing over this area loosens the underlying connective tissue, causing stretching and then redundancy (expansion) of the anal mucosa (inner lining). This force is greater when a small fecal bolus is pushed through an inadequately relaxed anus by raised intra-abdominal pressure alone.[3]

Dr. Tagart also tells us that the prolapse of the anal cushion begins above the pectinate line, or in the upper third of the anal canal. This explains why first- and second-degree hemorrhoids are distinguished by the purple mucosal lining of the anal canal. As the hemorrhoids expand, they will also protrude from the outer lining of the anal canal, which has the normal pinkish coloration.

Elastic Connective Tissue

Another English surgeon, Dr. W. H. F. Thomson, has conducted extensive research that confirms the importance of the elastic connective tissue which was emphasized in the above statement by Dr. Tagart.

After careful study of both normal and hemorrhoidal anal cushions, Dr. Thomson found that there was no significant difference between the tissue of the two cushions.[4] The structure of the blood vessels was also found to be quite similar. This particular finding is very important, as many medical references in the past have incorrectly stated that ". . . hemorrhoids are dilated veins of the anal canal or rectum."

Dr. Thomson concluded that hemorrhoids are simply displaced protrusions of the anal cushions, and these protrusions result from the breakdown of the supportive, elastic connective tissue.

The disruption of the elastic connective tissue was also noted by the American physicians Dr. O. C. Goss and Dr. J. Adams in 1950.[5] The longer the anal canal is subjected to the stress of passing stools of insufficient bulk, the more the connective tissue loses its elasticity and the greater will be the size of the developing hemorrhoid.

The elastic connective tissue of the anal canal can be compared to a rubber band. After ordinary stress it will readily return to its normal length. But if the elastic is required to undergo continual, excessive stretching, it gradually loses its flexibility. In the case of the anal connective tissue, it becomes less capable of anchoring the anal cushions to the internal sphincter muscles. The deterioration of the elastic connective tissue is followed by the displacement of the anal cushions.

At this time, medical research has not revealed which condition occurs first, the narrowing of the anal sphincters or the loss of elasticity of the anal connective tissue. It is likely that the two conditions develop simultaneously and work together to foster hemorrhoidal development.

THE HEMORRHOID

When the stool enters the constricted anal canal, which is swollen from the congested anal cushions, it is unable to progress without substantial straining by the patient. As the stool advances, it pushes the trapped blood ahead of it. This carries a portion of the cushions forward also, and after many prolonged periods of such straining, hemorrhoidal tissue may appear.

Initially, this displaced tissue consists of the lining of the anal canal, specifically the mucosal lining.[6] As the elasticity of the connective tissue continues to be impaired, a portion of the anal cushion beneath this mucosa also begins to bulge.

For most patients the progress of the developing hemorrhoid is a long steady course. It may be many years before dietary deficiencies and habitual straining cause the appearance of hemorrhoids. In a study of more than 23,000 patients with hemorrhoids, it was found that only eight percent were under thirty.[7] Many medical authorities believe that the development of hemorrhoids begins in the twenties. In my case, symptoms were apparent in the late teens. This study also revealed that the average age of the hemorrhoid patient is in the mid-forties for both men and women.

STAGES OF HEMORRHOIDS

There are four progressive stages in the development of hemorrhoids.

First Degree

The pressure of straining on the stool eventually will result in a slight swelling of the lining and cushion from the upper third of the anal canal. In this stage the swelling will not be physically noticed by the patient, although a physician can observe these swellings during an examination. The passage of hard stools may scrape this swelling with sufficient force to cause slight bleeding, which may be the patient's only hint that hemorrhoids are developing. Since anal bleeding can be the result of numerous other factors, only an examination can confirm hemorrhoids as the source of the bleeding.

Second Degree

Following an additional period of straining, a small portion of the mucosa—or mucosa and cushion—may protrude at the anus during the course of a bowel movement. At this stage the elastic connective tissue is still strong enough to draw the hemorrhoid back within the anus unassisted after the bowel movement has been completed. For this reason many patients are unaware of hemorrhoidal problems at this stage also.

It is at this point that the patient may first experience a painful blood clot on the circle of the anus. This is a symptom of hemorrhoids and is fully discussed in Chapter 4.

Third Degree

In the third stage the hemorrhoid remains in the prolapsed position at the conclusion of the bowel movement. The patient must manually (and carefully) return the protruding tissue within the anus. While prolapsed, the hemorrhoid causes a dull, aching, uncomfortable feeling.

Initially, the prolapsed hemorrhoid may consist of only the mucosal lining of the upper third of the anal canal. The mucosal hemorrhoids may appear at any position on the circle of the anus. Later the larger hemorrhoids consisting of anal cushion tissue also develop. These mature hemorrhoids characteristically appear at the three o'clock, seven o'clock, and eleven o'clock positions on the anal verge (viewed from standing position). These, of course, are the same positions in which the anal cushions are located within the anal canal.

Fourth Degree

At this point the large amount of hemorrhoidal tissue becomes very difficult or impossible to replace entirely within the anal opening. A permanent bulge at the anus occurs, which contributes to difficulty in having a bowel movement. The degree of discomfort increases considerably, becoming quite painful and debilitating in many cases. When the patient attempts to avoid additional discomfort by postponing bowel movements, the condition only worsens more rapidly. This is a miserable situation.

After fourth-degree hemorrhoids have developed, the patient may find it necessary to seek emergency medical assistance. If sufficient time is not available to locate a physician trained in cryotherapy, the patient may be forced to accept excisional surgery as a medical remedy. Of course, this is usually the least desirable alternative in terms of patient discomfort and post-operative complications.

Dr. Sanford Savin (author of the Foreword and Addendum) reports that even fourth-degree hemorrhoids can be effectively treated by the technique of cryosurgery.

COMPLICATIONS

The related problems which plague hemorrhoid sufferers are numerous and vary with each patient, according to the personal habits that led to the condition. A number of these complications are also considered *symptoms*, and therefore receive a more thorough discussion in Chapter 6.

Blood Clot

This complication can be extremely painful during its short duration. It occurs when one of the blood vessels of the anal canal expands or bursts under excessive pressure. When this wound occurs beneath the anal skin lining of the canal, it is noticeable immediately. The blood fills a grape-sized area beneath the anal lining and hardens (coagulates).

Blood clots are often misidentified as hemorrhoids by the afflicted patient. Their causes and suggested treatment are the subject of the next chapter.

Bleeding (Hemorrhaging)

The first bleeding the patient notices is usually due to the passage of hard, dehydrated stools through a congested anal canal. Whenever a stinging sensation is noticed during a bowel movement, the stools are likely to be stained with varying amounts of blood. The abrasions caused by this action will bleed more profusely as the hemorrhoidal tissue enlarges. Such bleeding usually subsides as soon as the prolapsed hemorrhoids are replaced within the anal canal.

In the process of replacing the hemorrhoids, the tender anal skin or mucosa may be abraded by rough handling, also resulting in slight bleeding. For this reason the use of moistened toilet paper is suggested during replacement.

Bleeding may also occur due to the presence of a *fissure* on the margin of the anus. A fissure is a slight crack in the skin, usually the result of the passage of hardened stools.

Whatever the cause, bleeding from the anus should always be considered a serious matter, and immediate medical attention is advised. Excessive bleeding can result in a state of anemia, in addition to mental distress. The proctologist can quickly and easily determine the origin of such bleeding.

Inconvenient Prolapse

After third-degree hemorrhoids have developed, there may be numerous occasions when they will not wait until a bowel movement occurs to prolapse. They may prolapse in the middle of a hike, a basketball game, a dance, or even while you are standing in a long line. On these occasions you must excuse yourself to seek the privacy of a rest room. When a private place is not available, you can expect to be very uncomfortable. You may be forced to sit or lie down for relief when you are unable to replace the protruding hemorrhoids.

When you do have an opportunity to tuck the hemorrhoids back in, you are well advised also to have a bowel movement since this need is probably the reason for your problem.

Eventually you may decide to attempt a bowel movement prior to engaging in physical activities. This can be a good idea, but only if the body is prepared to cooperate naturally. If the body is not yet prepared to provide a bowel movement, then this may only cause additional straining—exactly what you should avoid.

As will be discussed later in greater detail, not only should we take time to have a bowel movement when our body provides the appropriate signal, but we should be careful not to *force* a bowel movement prior to receiving this signal.

If necessary we should arrange our physical activities according to the anticipated requirements of our bodies. If this is not possible, then a rescheduling of eating habits can accomplish the same goal. As discussed earlier, we should consume our largest meal approximately thirty-six hours prior to a time that will normally be convenient for a bowel movement. *And* this meal should consist of healthy foods so the body can digest and outprocess the meal in the normal thirty-six hours.

False Urges

Another complication encountered during the third stage of hemorrhoidal development is uncertainty as to when the bowel movement has been completed. When hemorrhoids are in the prolapsed position, they may cause a sense of *fullness* within the anal canal and rectum, which encourages the patient to remain on the toilet. Continuing to strain is futile when the anal canal and rectum are already empty, in addition to being foolhardy at any time.

Being unable to distinguish between this false sensation and a genuine urge to defecate, we may strain to the extent that further hemorrhoidal development occurs. Under these circumstances, controlling bowel movements becomes "guess-work."

When the patient experiences this problem, the best course of action is to get off the toilet bowl quickly whenever there is any doubt as to the genuineness of the urge to push. It should be remembered that when a healthy diet is being consumed, it is seldom necessary to tarry longer than a minute or two on the toilet (once the movement has begun). So get off the toilet, tuck the hemorrhoids back in, and see if the urge doesn't fade away within a few minutes. You may be surprised how often you've wasted time and strained unnecessarily due to false urges caused by prolapsed hemorrhoids.

Strangulated Hemorrhoid

If the prolapsed hemorrhoidal tissue is not replaced relatively soon, as occasionally happens in the very young and elderly, the hemorrhoid may become strangulated. This problem arises when the external anal sphincter cuts off the blood supply of the prolapsed hemorrhoid over a lengthy period of time. This is a serious complication and requires immediate medical attention.

Skin Tags

These are often misidentified as "external hemorrhoids." They are actually small tags of skin located at the margin of the anus. Most often they are the remnants of either a blood clot or previous medical treatments for hemorrhoids.

When not kept scrupulously clean, skin tags can be a source of anal irritation and itching. If you have this problem, you should bathe more frequently, especially after bowel movements. When this is not possible, at least use moistened toilet paper, which provides a more thorough cleansing than dry paper.

Note to physicians: This book does not label hemorrhoids as external and internal. That an external hemorrhoid lies beneath internal tissue of the anal canal (the outer two-thirds) would certainly be confusing to a lay person, as would calling skin tags and permanently prolapsed hemorrhoidal tissue "external hemorrhoids." Non-physicians who do not understand this note need not be concerned.

Chapter 4

Blood Clots

The proper identification and treatment of blood clots is a controversial subject. British researchers, as typified by surgeon Dr. J. P. Partridge, unequivocally state that:

> . . . skin tags around the anus and a thrombosed perianal haematoma (blood clot) . . . are not hemorrhoids, and the use of the word "pile" in relation to them should be dropped.[1]

On the other hand, American researchers (in a study done at the Ferguson Clinic and reported by Dr. Mandel Ganchrow, et al.) report that on tissues from a hundred consecutive excisions, each case revealed that the blood clots were located within the hemorrhoidal tissues.[2] If this is the case, then the occurrence of the blood clot might be more accurately described as a complication of a hemorrhoidal condition, and many times it is the first warning sign.

The medical textbook *Diseases of the Colon and Anorectum* provides the following description of a blood clot:

> A thrombosed hemorrhoid is a hemorrhoid in which clotting of the blood has occurred. Its vessel wall may be intact and the clot confined entirely in its lumen. But

more often, the vein has ruptured and some blood has extravasated into the surrounding tissue to form a perivascular hematoma.[3]

Blood clots may appear at three different locations in the area of the anal canal:

1. beneath the modified anal skin (outer two-thirds of the anal canal),
2. beneath the mucosa (inner third of the anal canal), and
3. beneath skin which is wholly outside of the anus (within permanently prolapsed hemorrhoidal tissue).

Beneath Anal Skin

The type of blood clot most frequently experienced is one that develops beneath the modified anal skin (just within the anal opening). The swelling causes the clot to bulge outside of the anus. This bulge has the appearance of a firm grape, being tender to the touch and impossible to permanently tuck back within the anus. The swelling also smarts, the pain being somewhat similar to that of a large blood blister. This condition is often referred to as an "attack of hemorrhoids," or as a "swelling of hemorrhoidal tissues due to inflammation" in nonmedical publications.

Beneath Mucosa

When the blood clot occurs beneath the mucosa (mucous membrane) lining of the anal canal, it is rarely noticed due to the lack of sensitivity of this tissue.

Beneath External Skin

Blood clots may also appear in tissue which is completely outside of the anus. This is often the result of the prolapse of a strangulated internal hemorrhoid which obstructs the circulation, thereby causing clotting to occur in the adjacent external mass. This form of blood clot can be extremely painful and requires immediate medical attention.

A fair number of individuals who are afflicted with blood clots have not yet developed hemorrhoidal tissue that is evident to themselves. There are numerous persons in this category whom I have interviewed, and rarely do they believe that they also suffer from hemorrhoids.

Unfortunately for these individuals, the clinical evidence reported by Dr. Ganchrow strongly suggests that the blood clots discussed in this book are invariably associated with hemorrhoidal tissue.[4]

CAUSES

What the precise cause or causes of blood clots may be has yet to be determined. There are several possibilities.

Dr. J. C. Goligher, the author of *Surgery of the Anus, Rectum, and Colon,* states that blood clots are due to a prolapsed hemorrhoid being nipped by the external sphincter muscle of the anal canal, thereby rupturing a blood vessel.[5] The escaping blood then engorges the surrounding tissue, quickly hardening into a blood clot.

As noted earlier, blood clots may also appear beneath the mucosa of the anal canal where their term may pass completely unnoticed. These blood clots may be the result of a small hemorrhoid being pinched off by an exceptionally hard stool.

Dr. Tagart states that blood clots of the anus are caused by "dietary, and in particular, *alcoholic excess.*" [6] This statement coincides with the experiences of many persons I interviewed.

After the patient has developed more advanced hemorrhoids, excessive and lengthy straining during a bowel movement appears to be important as a cause of blood clots.

ONSET

When a fairly abrupt onset of pain occurs, accompanied by a swelling on the perimeter of the anus or within external tissue, a blood clot is the usual diagnosis. This swelling will be hard and tender to the touch. The first reaction of the patient, especially if third-degree hemorrhoids are present, is to attempt to replace this swelling within the anus. Usually this cannot be done with any permanence, and holding the blood clot within the anus does not result in a reduction of discomfort as in the case of a hemorrhoid. Instead such pressure only increases the discomfort.

TREATMENT

Bloods clots differ widely in size, intensity of pain, and location. In most cases the normal course of events will be that the clots will diminish of their own accord. If the pain and swelling are severe enough or persist, then medical attention should be sought. When the lump persists, even if it is no longer painful, the patient should also seek medical attention.

Personal

Medical references offer a wide variety of advice to the blood-clot victim. One suggests that some relief may be obtained by lying down with the hips elevated.[7] Another text suggests that one should go to bed, take oral analgesics (painkilers), lie prone with an icebag on the anus, use a stool softener, and drink no alcohol.[8] Some persons may find relief by gently massaging the clot while soaking in a tub of warm water. How well the above measures relieve discomfort will vary with the blood clot and the individual.

Natural Resolution

At the time that each of my blood clots occurred, I was unaware of the fact that the swelling and inflammation associated with most blood clots diminish of their own accord.

Dr. Robert T. Turell's *Diseases of the Colon and Anorectum* (Volume II, 1969) states:

> If untreated, the constant burning pain usually persists for five to seven days, diminishing gradually in intensity after the first day. If no further complications develop, the hard lump reaches its maximal size on the second day and thereafter slowly recedes, often leaving a hemorrhoidal skin tag as the residual. . . .[9]

According to Dr. Goligher's *Surgery of the Anus, Rectum, and Colon* (Second Edition, 1967):

> . . . the natural course of events in the majority of cases with this complication is spontaneous resolution.[10]

Medical

Readers should note the previous words of Dr. Turell: "If no further complications develop . . ." Such complications may include gangrenous tissue, bleeding, a fissure, infection, and a resultant abscess or fistula.[11]

Due to the intensity of the pain, many patients do not require any further encouragement to seek medical attention. Standard medical procedure is to excise (cut out) the clot, which requires only a minute or two, using a local anesthetic.

When the clot has occurred in external tissue, it may be necessary to remove this tissue entirely as it may not be possible to excise a single clot in such tissue.[12]

Injection is occasionally used to reduce the swelling and pain of minor blood clots, but this is not common practice.

One of the reasons may be that the swelling will usually return within twenty-four hours.[13]

The prescription of desensitizing ointments also has limited effectiveness, as the blood clot lies beneath the skin where ointments do not readily penetrate.[14]

The natural tendency of blood clots to undergo spontaneous resolution is exploited by commercial interests as we shall read later in this chapter and also in Chapter 11.

EXAMINATIONS

When the patient does make an appointment with a physician, it is important that the physician give due consideration to the discomfort of the hemorrhoid sufferer before conducting an examination with instruments.

My first experience in a proctologist's office was for the excision of a blood clot. Before the excision, a sigmoidoscopic exam was conducted which was quite discomforting (see Chapter 16 for a description of this type of examination). In contrast, years later when I had the same examination prior to cryotherapy, it was an acceptable, tolerable affair.

The skill and gentleness of the physician are quite important when examinations are conducted during the early course of a blood clot. Whether an examination should be conducted and by which instruments are decisions which the physician must evaluate in each individual case.

COMMERCIAL PRODUCTS

In seeking commercial ointments, salves, and other preparations to ease the pain or lubricate the anal canal, caution is advised.

Vasoconstrictors

One type of product deserves special attention in this regard. Any commercial product that contains *ephedrine* or *phenylephrine* may have the effect of aggravating the condition. The following is quoted from an official publication of the American Pharmaceutical Association:

> . . . the vasoconstrictors, including ephedrine and phenylephrine, are intended to reduce bleeding from hemorrhoids, but clinical evidence to support this claim is not available. They produce capillary and arteriole constrictions but their effect on veins is negligible.[15]

The advice of the editors of *Consumer Reports* is:

> The self-treatment of any of the various rectal or anal disorders with proprietary ointments or suppositories not only may aggravate the trouble and sensitize the skin, but may result in the overlooking of serious organic lesions.[16]

Until additional research determines that such products are safe, they should be used with caution or by direction of a physician.

THE GREAT HOAX

One commercial product promises to help "shrink and soothe swelling and inflamed hemorrhoidal tissue," while another such product advertises that it will "actually help shrink the swelling of hemorrhoidal tissue caused by inflammation." As a result, many persons who suffer from blood clots seek relief through the purchase of these products.

This advertising appears in virtually every form of the media—newspapers, magazines, television, and radio.

It is unfortunate that these advertisements do not state that blood clots will usually begin to lessen in severity *naturally* within forty-eight hours of their onset.

The pain generally begins to lessen after twenty-four hours and the swelling begins to subside after forty-eight hours.[17]

When the blood clot becomes less painful and begins to shrink in size of its own accord, these persons may incorrectly attribute their relief to the purchase of the advertised commercial products. This hoax helps foster an industry which reportedly grossed more than forty million dollars in 1973.[18]

The best treatment for blood clots will vary with each patient, depending on the nature of the clot and the degree of discomfort experienced. When the patient is not excessively bothered by the pain, conservative treatment as mentioned earlier in the chapter may suffice. A reclining position, warm baths, the use of icebags, and engaging in distracting activities may provide adequate relief.

If these measures seem insufficient, the physician requires little more than a minute to excise the clotted blood in most cases. The resulting wound will usually hurt less than the clot, but some discomfort may continue for a few more days.

The use of drugs should be by direction of a physician, after a review of your condition.

A benefit of seeking medical advice at this time is that the physician can determine the degree of hemorrhoidal development and provide information which may assist in halting further development.

Chapter 5

What Causes Hemorrhoids?

The following discussion between two physicians occurred during a symposium presented at the American Proctologic Society in 1972:

> Dr. Terrell: Dr. Ferguson, do you try to find the cause of hemorrhoids in all cases you see and operate upon?
> Dr. Ferguson: Do we find a cause?
> Dr. Terrell: Do you search for a cause for hemorrhoids?
> Dr. Ferguson: No.[1]

Only a few years earlier, Dr. Terrell had written in the *American Journal of Surgery:*

> Investigations of the cause of hemorrhoidal disorders have remained controversial or inconclusive (a conclusion in which nothing is concluded). In view of this limited knowledge of the cause, therapy leaves much to be desired. In a past editorial, it was stated that the management of piles may be effected by three alternate methods: They may be neglected, injected, or resected.[2]

Fortunately, there has been a considerable amount of attention given to this subject in European medical circles.

DISPELLING A FEW MYTHS

The vision of many medical authorities is often limited to the experience they've gained within their own societies. When these societies have been confined to those of the Western industrialized nations, it has encouraged the acceptance of a number of "myths" which should be disposed of before we begin a discussion of the causes of hemorrhoids.

Man's Upright Position and Lack of Valves in the Portal Veins

Many medical publications today insist that man's upright position and the absence of valves in the veins of the portal system (leading from the rectum to the liver) are leading causes for the development of hemorrhoids. If these two universal human characteristics were prime causes of this condition, we might expect to find a high incidence of hemorrhoids in the populations of all nations.

In fact, we seldom find hemorrhoids among the rural populations of the relatively undeveloped nations of Asia, Africa, and South America.[3] Instances of this affliction are quite rare among these peoples, comprising the vast majority of the world's population.

Of course, the populations of these nonindustrialized nations walk in upright positions just as we do, and their portal veins also lack valves. Therefore, it is quite obvious that these two factors cannot be the causes of hemorrhoids.

Medical authorities who propound these false theories do a disservice to their patients and their profession. When one accepts such erroneous ideas, then it is too easy to assume that the development of hemorrhoids is inevitable. Believing this, many persons might assume that there is little to be done in order to prevent their occurrence—a conclusion which is *totally* inaccurate.

Age

This factor is also frequently suggested as a cause of hemorrhoids, with equally poor justification.

Modern medical texts now suggest that people first develop hemorrhoids in their twenties or thirties, primarily due to an "accumulation of sins," rather than to reaching a certain age level.[4] If attaining a particular age level were really a cause of hemorrhoids, then everyone over that level would have hemorrhoids. But this is not the case, since many persons are free of this affliction all of their lives. Again the persons in underdeveloped nations over a certain age might also be expected to have hemorrhoids and they do not.

Heredity

The prevalence of hemorrhoids in a particular family is usually due to similar dietary and personal habits, rather than inherited physical characteristics.[5] The initial toilet training which children receive has much to do with their poor toilet habits in later life. This should not be considered a hereditary factor; instead, it is usually the result of inexperienced parents.

Miscellaneous

Coughing, sneezing, vomiting, horseback riding, pregnancy, sitting on hot radiators (believe it or not), prolonged standing, erect posture, and a host of other reasons are often blamed in medical texts for the development of hemorrhoids. All these factors also occur in developing nations and do not lead to hemorrhoids (although I'm not sure they sit on hot radiators in developing nations).

PERSONAL CONSIDERATIONS

Precisely why a person develops hemorrhoids depends upon the particular habits of that individual.

If one's purpose in reviewing this chapter is to discover why hemorrhoids have developed, then it is necessary to examine the following information in the light of one's own habits.

In some cases hemorrhoidal development may be primarily due to dietary factors; while in other instances the main causes may be cultural factors, such as childhood toilet training or the limiting circumstances of social and job requirements. In the majority of cases though, we will probably find that *both* dietary and cultural habits have played a role in the development of hemorrhoids.

Dietary Factors

Eating habits are considered the most important factor for several reasons:

1. If the diet is the leading cause of one's hemorrhoidal development, then only an improvement in this diet will provide a significant benefit.
2. An improved diet may partially compensate for adverse social or working conditions which are beyond the individual's immediate control.
3. Dietary habits are easier to alter than personal habits which have developed and existed over a period of many years.

Cultural Factors

Although these are usually of secondary importance, poor personal habits can frustrate efforts to improve a hemorrhoidal condition simply because habits can be so difficult to change. Changing one's habits involves a relearning process which requires time, discipline, and practice.

The most serious habit which requires relearning is the tendency to postpone normal bowel functioning. The need for a bowel movement should be fulfilled while the body's signal is still strong. Habitual postponing of bowel movements can lead to serious consequences, including:

1. loss of the rectal reflex, requiring undesirable straining to accomplish elimination, and
2. hardening of the feces, as the longer they remain within the bowels unnecessarily, the less moisture they retain.

STRAINING, THE MAJOR CAUSE

After reading the three preceding chapters, you should be aware that the major causative factor in the development of the hemorrhoidal cushion is straining while on the toilet.

This straining is usually the result of constipation.[6] A person becomes constipated due to the previously discussed:

1. dietary factors,
2. poor personal habits, or
3. related illnesses.

The British surgeons, Denis P. Burkitt and C. W. Graham-Stewart, prominent in the field of intestinal disorders, tell us:

> . . . the direct cause is believed to be raised intra-abdominal pressure effected by straining to evacuate *hard stools*.[7]

Hard stools, like small stools, are a common symptom of the state of constipation.

Dr. Tagart tells us:

> . . . hemorrhoids are caused by straining to force an unnaturally small stool through the anal canal rather

> than allowing the stimulated rectal muscles to expel one of four centimeters or more in diameter.[8]

The quantity and quality of one's stools are strongly influenced by dietary factors and, to a lesser degree, by one's personal habits.

Medical authorities, in increasing numbers, believe that the modern approach to solving medical problems is to study healthy bodies which are functioning properly. By studying what provides the body protection from disease, it is much easier to determine what has malfunctioned within the body.

Using this approach, we must study people who are free of hemorrhoids. Fortunately, we have available for such study whole societies that are free of hemorrhoids.

THE PECULIAR ELEMENT OF DIET

In countries where the occurrence of hemorrhoids is rare, we find a number of dietary elements which are uncommon in the highly industrialized societies of the Western world. One of these elements seems to be very important in determining why the digestive tract can function properly and efficiently.

Dr. Joseph Franklin Montague, author of *The Modern Treatment of Hemorrhoids* (written fifty years ago) observed:

> . . . that men accustomed to living in a rough, primeval life involving considerable muscular activity, as well as the subsistence on a coarse diet, are rarely troubled with this condition.[9]

This is not to suggest that we must return to caves or the trees to hunt for our own foods. We need hunt no farther than the nearest supermarket for "coarse" foods. These are plant foods in which the skin, inner fiber, and/or residue have not been filtered (refined) out. Among those who are health conscious, it is becoming popular to add this coarseness (dietary fiber) back into our diets in the form of unprocessed miller's bran.

Of the many available words describing this peculiar element—husk, skin, fiber, residue, and roughage—we shall use "fiber" in the balance of this book.

In an article appearing in the *Postgraduate Medical Journal* of September, 1975, Drs. Burkitt and Graham-Stewart tell us:

> The fundamental cause of constipation is held to be the large proportion of calories consumed in the Western world in the form of fiber-depleted carbohydrate foods and of white flour and sugar in particular.[10]

Dr. Burkitt has spent twenty years practicing medicine in Africa, and considerably more time conducting medical research concerning the population on this continent. His studies include the results of statistics gathered at more than one hundred hospitals of twenty African nations.[11]

The gathering of monthly statistics at seventy-three of the above-mentioned hospitals revealed that each hospital saw an average of less than three patients per year in which the ailment was diagnosed as hemorrhoids. This is in contrast to the hospitals of the United States, where the hemorrhoidectomy has been one of the most frequently performed hospital operations.[12]

Dr. Burkitt also determined that rural people in these underdeveloped nations consumed large amounts of "*lightly processed carbohydrate foods rich in plant fiber.*" This resulted in larger and softer stools, in addition to a shorter transit time in comparison with the results of the typical Western diet of "refined carbohydrate foods depleted in fiber." *Transit time* refers to the time required to ingest and eliminate food matter.

Dr. Burkitt established a very definite relationship between the fiber content of food, the speed of intestinal transit, and the weight and consistency of stools.

His comparisons between the results of diets consumed by English schoolboys and a group of African villagers were dramatic. Whereas the schoolboys on a normal, refined English diet passed an average daily stool of 108 grams, the African villagers on an unrefined diet passed an average daily stool of 400 grams.[13]

The average transit time of the English schoolboys was seventy-seven hours, and the average transit time for the Africans was thirty-five hours.[14]

Another well-known British physician, Dr. Neil S. Painter, reports that:

> . . . the average daily stool in England and the United States is less than 150 grams, and food residue may take up to five days to pass from the mouth to the anus; these stiff stools often are voided only with effort.

He goes on to reveal that the typical Ugandan villager:

> . . . passes about 450 grams of moist stool daily without any significant effort and with a food residue transit time of less than 35 hours.[15]

Some people might suppose that their digestive systems could not possibly function with the same smoothness and efficiency as that of an African villager.

Additional research by Dr. Painter has revealed:

> The addition of fiber in the form of unprocessed bran to the diet of British patients results in stool weights and transit times very similar to those of African villagers.[16]

The incidence of hemorrhoids in Africans has been low, in the experience of many other British doctors. At the Charles Johnson Memorial Hospital in Zululand (Republic of South Africa), of 100,000 patients seen over a three-year period of time, only one had hemorrhoids.[17]

Dr. Hugh S. Trowell relates his experiences by telling us:

> He had seen only two cases of anemia due to bleeding piles in 30 years in East Africa, and one was a prince on a semi-European diet.[18]

Nigeria is one of the African nations that have been heavily influenced by the culture of "Western civilization," and therefore has a greater incidence of hemorrhoidal disease than other "less-developed" African nations.[19]

The summary of a seven-year study conducted by Dr. O. O. Ajayi, a physician in Nigeria, reviews the case histories of three hundred hemorrhoid patients admitted to the University College Hospital in Ibadan, West Nigeria. This summary reveals:

> Increasing sophistication and changing food habits in the cities and towns and the attendant limitations on defecating at will are suggested as responsible etiologic (causative) factors.[20]

Affluence and Fiber-Depleted Diets

With increasing affluence, man seems to prefer the more expensive foods which are available to him. These foods in most societies are refined carbohydrates and the *high-protein animal products.* Frequently these foods are consumed to the exclusion of the less expensive natural grains and fresh fruits and vegetables. In the economically emerging nations, this pattern of dietary change has been accompanied by a corresponding increase in hemorrhoids.[21,22,23,24]

In discussing the occurrence of hemorrhoids, Dr. Tagart reports:

> The incidence rises with the progressive refining of cereals to eliminate the husk and as the proportion of meat-derived protein in the diet increases.[25]

Particular note should be given to the portion of the above statement which refers to the *consumption of meat-derived protein.*

A few medical references refer to the relatively high incidence of hemorrhoids in middle-aged professional athletes. It is generally known that athletes and would-be athletes are encouraged to consume large portions of meat, milk, and other animal-protein products. Instead of attributing the development of hemorrhoids in athletes to greater physical activity, it may be more accurate to consider their diets as the major causative factor.

Roller Mills and Related Illnesses

There was a time, not long ago, when hemorrhoids were fairly uncommon, even in Western cultures. With the introduction of steel roller mills in the 1880's, the fiber content of flour was greatly reduced.

Fiber is refined out of many foods for various reasons, but primarily for the convenience of the consumer and profit of the food industry. Without its fiber a food is easier to chew and therefore can be swallowed quicker. In a given period of time, an individual eating refined foods can consume considerably more in volume than another individual eating unrefined foods. Food manufacturers and retailers quickly realize the economics of this difference and take advantage of it.

The proper mastication of foods causes the secretion of a quart of juices within the mouth and two quarts of gastric juices in the stomach during the course of one day. When food is refined to eliminate the need for much of this chewing, it also eliminates a large percentage of gastric and digestive juices that would normally flow into the stomach. Without the proper flow of these juices into the stomach, a person does not reach a sense of fullness as quickly. This also explains why a person can consume a greater volume of fiber-depleted foods. And it explains many cases of obesity.

Food fiber has several qualities which should be clearly understood:

1. It is not digested, but passes through the body essentially unchanged.
2. This fiber has an ability to absorb and retain moisture during its passage through the digestive tract.

When a person consumes a meal with plenty of fiber, the stomach will be partially filled with matter which is never digested. There is nothing wrong with this; as a matter of fact, it is absolutely essential that this indigestible food matter be present. The function of the fiber is to ensure that all foods entering the digestive system remain moist during their transit through the body.

This moistness facilitates the movement of food matter along the lengthy gastrointestinal passages. Peristalsis can more effectively move food matter which has been lubricated with moisture. The presence of the undigested food fiber also provides the necessary bulk to the stools, so the rectal reflex can be properly stimulated.

A diet that is low in fiber has been found to be of prime importance in the development of other illnesses.

These include:

1. Anal fissures (cracks) and fistulas (abscesses) [26]
2. Varicose veins [27]
3. Deep vein thrombosis [28]
4. Embolisms (obstruction of blood vessel by a clot) [29]
5. Appendicitis [30]
6. Diverticular disease [31]
7. Hiatus hernia [32]
8. Arteriosclerosis [33]
9. Ischemic heart disease (temporary lack of blood supply) [34]
10. Coronary thrombosis [35]
11. Diabetes *mellitus* [36]
12. Cancer of the colon [37]
13. Cancer of the rectum.[38]

Hemorrhoids are a sign or symptom that there is something seriously wrong with one's diet. Hemorrhoids can also be a forewarning that unless the diet is subtantially improved, a far more serious physical ailment may yet develop.

CONTRIBUTING CULTURAL FACTORS

Hemorrhoids are sometimes referred to as the "disease of civilization."

The pressure and requirements of conforming to the 'needs' of modern society often encourage many serious physical disorders, of which hemorrhoids are one of the first to appear.

This "civilizing" of a society results in a number of significant changes in daily activity which are conducive to hemorrhoids. A few of the more important changes are:

1. a tendency to postpone bowel movements beyond reasonable limits,
2. attempts to change natural toilet habits to a demand basis,
3. devotion of less time to physical activities necessary to maintain good health,
4. indulging frequently to excess in food and drink, and
5. the use of laxatives in an attempt to regain lost regularity of toilet habits.

Postponing Needed Bowel Movements

When the rectal reflex (urge) is initiated, we all-too-often find it is not convenient to go to the toilet. We may be in a rush to get dressed or on our way to work, and once at our job it may be necessary to wait until the midmorning break. By that time the urge may be gone.

The rectal reflex is usually initiated by the peristalsis that follows a meal. When dinner guests are present or when we are dining out, it may not be convenient to find relief if an urge for a bowel movement occurs. It is perfectly natural that most people desire a quiet place of privacy at this time, and, consequently, they may wait until the middle of the day or even the end of the day before having a bowel movement that should have occurred in the morning.

Clinical experience has determined that if the bowel movement does not follow the rectal reflex, the urge may fade away and not return again until after another meal fills the stomach.[39] When a person attempts to have a bowel movement without a strong rectal reflex to initiate the elimination, straining may be necessary.

During the period of time that the stool remains in the rectum or lower colon unnecessarily, this congestion causes two problems:

1. the longer the fecal matter remains in this area the *less moist* it becomes and therefore more difficult to eliminate, and
2. the pressure of the congestion on the wall of the rectum tends to inhibit the natural flow of blood from the anal canal (the portal veins pass through the muscles in the wall of the rectum).[40]

When the stools have dried out substantially and are quite hard, their elimination can cause slight bleeding. This often occurs during the early stages of hemorrhoidal development, as well as later.

The regular inhibition of the rectal reflex can also result in progressively weaker signals to the rectum during peristalsis.[41] Eventually it may become difficult to naturally eliminate proper stools without some straining, simply because the rectal reflex has been so weakened. This reflex is not unlike a body muscle which becomes weak through lack of use. Once the rectal reflex has been ignored long enough, its weakened state may make it quite difficult for the patient to determine when a bowel movement is needed.

Dr. G. C. Prasad of India reported in the June, 1976, issue of the *American Journal of Proctology* that after investigating the habits of 123 patients with hemorrhoids, it was found that 67 percent of the cases "showed habits of withholding the natural urges." [42]

Occupations

As mentioned earlier, many people find it impossible to follow their body's natural urges due to the nature of their employment. West Coast stockbrokers seem to have a high incidence of the affliction, which may be accounted for by the opening time of the stock market—7:00 A.M., West Coast time. Jobs which require early morning starting times often leave little time for proper nutrition or toilet habits.

Pilots also seem to be prone to hemorrhoids, probably due to the relative rigidity of their jobs.

Letter carriers frequently suffer such problems, possibly due to the lack of facilities on many postal routes.

Any job which ties the worker to a desk or machine for unvarying periods of time can inhibit natural functioning.

Sitting Style

Parents in the Western world generally keep their babies diapered at all times. When the parents decide that it is time to toilet train their child, it is often a traumatic experience for the baby. After years of defecating at will, the baby must learn to reverse its natural instinct and defecate at its *parents'* will.

There is only one way to do this. Unless the parents' timing is intelligently planned, the baby must learn to strain. It is easy to understand why a parent tires of cleaning messy diapers, not to mention the messy baby. But the child may have difficulty understanding that straining is necessary to satisfy the parent. The difficulties of the child are often compounded by parents who feed the baby foods that are constipating. It does not take long for a child to learn the habit of straining under such circumstances.

In many homes the bathroom is considered the library or "reading room." Dr. Goligher declares:

> Faulty habits of defecation can be equally bad, for some individuals instead of having a smooth, easy daily motion lasting at most a few minutes, indulge in an orgy of protracted straining at the stool, interspersed with reading of the morning paper.[43]

In *Understanding Surgery*, a book written for the general public by Dr. Robert E. Rothenberg, we are told:

> Irregularity of bowel evacuation, prolonged sojourns upon the toilet, and chronic constipation are contributors toward their formation.[44]

This comment appears in a section concerning abdominal surgery as it relates to hemorrhoids.

Lack of Exercise

Many people are unaware that it is primarily muscular action of the body which causes the blood in our veins to return to the heart. Without some form of daily exercise, our circulation can become quite sluggish. The body can be compared to a motor vehicle which also suffers if its activity is confined to short "stop-and-go" motion. In order for a car to stay well tuned, regular use at cruising speeds is necessary. For our bodies this means sufficient physical action to get the blood moving *briskly*.

Dr. Montague stated fifty years ago:

> Muscular action is efficient in preventing this condition (hemorrhoids) in two ways; first by raising the physiological requirement for food so that overeating does not occur so readily; and second, and more important, is the fact that in a life of muscular activity there is no chance for portal plethora or venous engorgement elsewhere in the body.[45]

The last portion of Montague's statement refers directly to the quality of circulation in the veins leading from the anal canal to the liver.

Dr. Marion C. Pruitt, author of the medical text *Hemorrhoids,* goes so far as to suggest:

> Change in occupation may be necessary when the patient leads a sedentary life or has irregular habits with little or no exercise.[46]

Orgies

Among the twenty-six causes of hemorrhoids listed in one reference were "passions" and "obesity." [47]

The excess consumption of alcoholic beverages is mentioned by numerous medical authorities as responsibile for the onset of hemorrhoids, especially the blood clots associated with the condition.

Dr. Montague states:

> Indeed, a careful history will, in many instances, show that an orgy of eating or drinking preceded the attack for which the patient presents himself to the physician.[48]

In the medical text *Diseases of the Colon and Anorectum* (Volume II) a physician notes:

> I have observed for a number of years two patients who indulge in repeated bouts of excessive drinking to a degree sufficient to produce a presumed alcoholic hepatitis manifested by a transient but marked enlargement of the liver . . . in both patients their long-existing hemorrhoids became enlarged and symptomatic during these periods of hepatomegaly and recede appreciably as the liver returns nearly to its normal size and function.[49]

That we practice moderation in the consumption of food and drink is common sense, yet many people make it a contest to see how much they can consume or drink in one session. Among the problems which may result, hemorrhoids are quite common.

Laxatives

Contrary to popular belief, laxatives are a major cause of constipation.[50] As such, they may also be considered a prime factor in the development of hemorrhoids.

The following statement is quoted from the medical textbook *The Modern Treatment of Hemorrhoids* (1926):

> One of the most flagrant, if not the most frequent, exciting causes of hemorrhoid formation is the abuse of cathartics (laxatives). Self-medication has, however, because of insistent advertising suggestions, become so universal, particularly in respect to cathartics, that a very considerable percentage of people are victims of this habit. Since it leads to further constipation, and is productive of much local mucosal irritation and congestion, there is but little doubt as to its role in hemorrhoidal production. In the instance of some of the more irritating cathartics, they may actually be the primary cause of hemorrhoidal formation.[51]

Additional information on this subject is provided in a chapter devoted to laxatives.

Pregnancy

The state of pregnancy deserves discussion at this point as many people, including physicians, believe that it is a major contributing factor in the formation of hemorrhoids. This is not totally accurate. Recent research findings suggest that the woman who experiences hemorrhoids during the latter stages of pregnancy probably had them prior to becoming pregnant. The presence of the increased abdominal pressure simply causes the hemorrhoids to become more symptomatic.

A study of the causes of hemorrhoids conducted by Dr. Lyon Hyams and Dr. John Philpot, members of the Rutgers Medical School, found that the onset of hemorrhoids in pregnant women is precipitated where the woman is susceptible.[52] Such women may have had first- or second-degree hemorrhoids prior to pregnancy, the hemorrhoids quickly reaching the *prolapsing* third-degree stage when the women attain full term.

We are told in *Diseases of the Colon and Anorectum* that it is not uncommon for a pregnant woman "to develop" mild hemorrhoids during the latter months of pregnancy, and that it is also common for them to dissipate and disappear within three months after delivery.[53]

In countries where the majority of the population subsists on a high-fiber diet, hemorrhoids are rarely a complication of pregnancy.[54] This suggests that the dietary habits of women in the Western world may be more important in the appearance of hemorrhoids during the period of pregnancy than the state of pregnancy itself.

Related Illnesses

There are many related illnesses of the body which are said to be contributory to hemorrhoids. Of these, cancer of the rectum is the most serious. When this disease occurs, it causes a sense of fullness within the rectum which encourages unnecessary straining by the patient.

An article appearing in the February, 1976, issue of *Diseases of the Colon and Anorectum* reveals:

> Recently, cancer of the colon and rectum has been suggested to be significantly related to dietary content, unduly prolonged intestinal transit time, and bowel habits.[55]

Enlargement of the liver has already been discussed as a cause of additional blood pressure within the cushions of the anal canal. Alcoholic excesses lead to this condition frequently.

The numerous diseases which interfere with normal digestion also cause problems in elimination. Dietary factors appear to be quite important in the development of most of these diseases. When the obsession in the Western world to have a daily bowel movement is combined with the generally constipating diets of many people, hemorrhoids are the inevitable result.

Chapter 6

Symptoms

The most common symptoms of hemorrhoids are bleeding and prolapse. Blood clots are an infrequent indication. There is a great variety of opinion concerning which symptom should appear first. A slight majority of medical opinion states that bleeding might occur first, although many people seem to experience either prolapse or a blood clot initially.

Which symptom occurs first is determined by the particular habits of each individual. When dietary habits lead to constipating hard stools, their harsh scraping action encourages bleeding when hemorrhoids are developing.

When faulty toilet habits result in habitual, prolonged straining, the eventual prolapse of hemorrhoidal tissue may occur first.

Frequently it is difficult to determine which symptom appeared originally. Many people (80 percent in one study) do not seek a doctor's advice during the first twelve months after first noticing a symptom.[1] Thirty percent do not seek medical advice during the first ten years of a hemorrhoidal condition. After that length of time, many patients simply cannot recall which of their symptoms occurred first.

In any case, the question of which symptom should appear initially is not as important as the necessity that the patient seek immediate medical advice upon noticing *any* symptom.

WHY PATIENTS AVOID MEDICAL ATTENTION

Unfortunately, most people do not seek medical advice after noticing symptoms suggesting the presence of hemorrhoids. The reasons that people procastinate are varied, but the basic reasons seem to be:

1. embarrassment or a strong sense of privacy concerning the problem, and
2. a fear that the symptom may be a sign of a more serious disorder of the intestinal tract.

Inhibition

This book can do little to dispel a patient's sense of privacy in these matters other than to repeat that most hemorrhoid sufferers feel the same way—we have lots of company.

Studies by insurance companies in the early 1940's revealed that when the population of the United States numbered 140 million, a total of 25 million people had either had a hemorrhoidectomy or would require such treatment at sometime during their lifetimes.[2] The population of the United States has grown more than 50 percent since that time, suggesting that the number of serious hemorrhoid sufferers may now exceed 40 million.

Interestingly, I have found that almost all persons afflicted with hemorrhoids are willing to discuss their problem once another person has "broken the ice." Open, frank discussions of the nature and treatment of the condition can do much to reduce normal hesitation to seek proper medical care.

Fear of More Serious Disorder

Many patients, believing that hemorrhoidal symptoms *such as bleeding* are a sign of a more serious disorder, are afraid to confront a physician with their problem. The cumbersome, uncomfortable physical examinations of the lower bowels have also discouraged many patients from seeking proper care.

A STOOL TEST

Hemorrhoidal bleeding is normally noticed on the surface of the feces or on the cleansing tissue at the conclusion of the bowel movement. The blood is also bright red, being fresh.

Bleeding from sources other than hemorrhoids is characterized by blood within the feces, which is generally concealed from view. When blood is found within the feces, it may indicate a number of intestinal disorders, including:

1. ulcers,
2. diverticulosis (abnormal sacs of the lower intestine),
3. an esophageal varix (swollen vein),
4. a malignancy,
5. a primary blood disease, and
6. a number of other minor disorders.[3]

Medical research has recently developed a simple test to detect bleeding in the area of the intestinal tract above the anal canal.[4] It is quite similar to a urine test.

The stool test requires the patient to take a sample smear of the feces on three consecutive days, which can be done in the privacy of one's own home. The test kit is then returned to the physician's office, where a thirty-second chemical test is conducted to find evidence of concealed blood within the feces. There are a number of different names given to this test, of which a few are:

1. occult (concealed) blood test,
2. hemoccult (or hemacult) slide test,
3. guiac paper test, or
4. stool test.

Whatever name is used, the test is an effective means of detecting concealed blood within the feces, which indicates bleeding above the anal canal.

At a one-day mass screening in 1976, this test was given to 3,400 persons. The test turned up five unsuspected cases of colon and rectal cancers (among other disorders) which might have been untreated otherwise.[5] The American Cancer Society estimates that 75 percent of the victims of these forms of cancer could be saved if the disease were detected in its early stages.

Within the next few years, the stool test should become a standard part of all medical examinations. When the physician does not offer this test, the patient should request it.

With such a simple test available, patients should not hesitate to dispel their fears of having a more serious intestinal disorder when bleeding is noticed. Rectal bleeding is a signal for the patient to seek prompt medical assistance in order to diagnose the source. Physicians desiring technical information concerning this test should contact:

Smith Kline Diagnostics
Attention: Product Manager
800 Maude Ave.
Sunnyvale, Calif. 94086

BLEEDING—A MAJOR SYMPTOM

If bleeding is not the first symptom noticed by a hemorrhoid sufferer, it is still the first noticeable symptom. It may occur while the hemorrhoids are in the first stage of development; whereas the prolapse of hemorrhoidal tissue does not occur until the second and third stages of development.

Bleeding associated with hemorrhoids may vary in frequency and intensity, according to the size of the hemorrhoids and the hardness of the stools. Such bleeding is seldom painful, although a slight stinging may be felt as a hard stool scrapes a hemorrhoid, and may go unnoticed unless the patient is specifically watching for it.

On occasion, heavy bleeding can lead to anemia,[6] and may be accompanied by a feeling of lethargy, listlessness, and exhaustion even upon slight exertion. One's mental distress may also be increased.

PROLAPSE—A MAJOR SYMPTOM

Hemorrhoids do *not* appear suddenly. Many patients mistake the sudden appearance of a blood clot for hemorrhoids, since they are both characterized by a protrusion of tissue at the margin of the anus. The difference between a blood clot and a hemorrhoid is pain. The blood clot will be quite painful, while the new hemorrhoid will be only slightly uncomfortable until it is replaced.

The initial prolapse of hemorrhoidal tissue will be a small lump of the mucosal lining of the anal canal. As has been mentioned earlier, this lining has a purplish color and is relatively insensitive. During the second stage of hemorrhoidal development, this protrusion returns of its own accord within the anus at the conclusion of the bowel movement.

As the hemorrhoids are permitted or encouraged to grow, a larger lump the size of a medium-sized grape will begin to protrude during bowel movements. At this point in the growth of hemorrhoidal tissue, a portion of the anal cushion will also begin to protrude. These larger hemorrhoids will appear on the circle of the anus at the three, seven, and eleven o'clock positions (viewed from the rear with the patient standing).

When prolapse is first noticed, it is not painful, although it can be slightly discomforting. This discomfort increases as the hemorrhoids grow. Continual straining on the toilet and deficient dietary habits will eventually cause the hemorrhoidal tissue to remain in the prolapsed position at the conclusion of the bowel movement. With very large third-degree hemorrhoids, the accompanying discomfort may border on pain, especially during replacement.

Replacement

The patient should replace these third-degree hemorrhoids within the anal canal *with care.* The prolapsed tissue can be easily abraded during its replacement, causing irritation and bleeding.

The patient should exercise discretion in the use of commercially advertised lubricants, as such products can leave a residue of oil on the anal tissue. This oil not only collects undesirable matter but also inhibits its removal. The end result is often an uncomfortable itch.

Water or, in its absence, one's own saliva is the best lubricant to use when replacing hemorrhoids within the anal canal. To safely and smoothly return the prolapsed tissue, simply moisten a part of the toilet-tissue pad before applying pressure.

The patient will also find that moistened toilet tissue is superior to dry toilet tissue in the general cleaning of the anal area.

TREATING SYMPTOMS

When the patient uses commercially advertised preparations in an effort to treat hemorrhoids and other rectal ailments, only the symptoms receive treatment, however poor. A hemorrhoidal problem is probably due to a combination of poor toilet habits and a dietary deficiency leading to constipation, both of which are unaffected by commercial preparations.

Again, it is stressed that the patient seek prompt medical care for all rectal complaints. Consideration should also be given to the many causes of anorectal ailments, which have been discussed in the preceding chapter.

PART II

Personal Treatment

Chapter 7

Bran, the Miracle Fiber

For thousands of years, man has altered cereal grains in an effort to chew these foods more easily. In Roman times, as now, people have also equated whiteness in their foods with "purity." Entire industries have been developed to refine food for the physical and visual convenience of the consumer. In recent times (within the last one hundred years), the ability to refine sources of food energy has made especially rapid progress.

This progress has been accompanied by the emergence of a large number of diseases which had been considered quite rare before this century. Among these illnesses are peptic ulcers; arteriosclerosis; coronary thrombosis; pulmonary embolism; diabetes; appendicitis; cancer of the colon, rectum, and anal canal; diverticular disorders; varicose veins; deep vein thrombosis; hemorrhoids; and many others.[1,2,3]

It has only been within the last few years that the medical profession has given serious and wide attention to one of the basic causes of the above-listed illnesses—the Western "civilized" diet.[4] Prior to this time, modern medicine has been preoccupied with treating the symptoms of these illnesses.

In countries where medical care is provided equally to all citizens, we have seen serious concerted efforts to identify the causes of many illnesses. This emphasis on preventive medicine is necessitated not only by good sense, but by the economics of providing national medical care. We are fortunate to have available the research and experience of many medical professionals in these countries. They have found a solution to many intestinal disorders that is so simple that it almost defies common belief.

This chapter will discuss the manner in which the addition of *bran* to our diets can rapidly correct many of the irregularities and other difficulties that the body experiences during digestion and elimination.

WHAT IS BRAN?

A kernel of wheat is composed of three parts:

1. the heart of the kernel (the endosperm, 83 percent),
2. the embryo (the germ, 3 percent), and
3. the outer protective layers (the bran, 14 percent).[5]

The germ and bran are separated from the endosperm in the making of refined white flour. After separation, the wheat germ and bran are usually sold to the processors of livestock and poultry feeds.[6] There are some "good" reasons why the wheat germ and bran are separated and sold to the manufacturers of animal feeds.

Most persons in civilized societies do not feel that they are missing anything when their flour products no longer contain the wheat germ and bran. The majority of people seem to prefer their foods in an easily chewable form and with a pleasing white appearance. In the production of macaroni, spaghetti, and other pasta products, freedom from bran eliminates the appearance of specks.

The refined-food manufacturers are quite willing to accommodate these preferences, as they can then sell the germ and bran to animal and poultry-feed processors—thereby making an extra profit on the same amount of raw material. It is also a fact that when the wheat germ is left in the flour the shelf life of the product is thereby reduced. This, of course, would act to restrict profits and is considered undesirable by the food manufacturers.

The reasons that animal-feed processors purchase the "left-overs" from refining the wheat kernel is revealed in the following statement:

> . . . wheat bran, which people formerly ate, is now fed to domestic animals, because they can't stay fit without it.[7]

As it turns out, the human body does not stay fit without bran either.

The broken coat of the seed of other cereal grains is also considered bran. This fiber may be broken down into three basic components:

1. lignin (9 percent),
2. cellulose (40 percent), and
3. hemicelluloses (50 percent) and moisture (1 percent).[8]

The cellulose and hemicellulose components of bran have the ability to absorb large amounts of water. A portion of the hemicellulose actually becomes slippery when moistened.

FUNCTION OF BRAN

On the wheat kernel the primary function of the bran is to protect the seed from the elements until the proper temperature and moisture stimulate the growth of the seed.

In the human body the bran also plays a protective role. The presence of adequate bran in one's diet insures that the stools will be of proper consistency and volume to pass smoothly through the small intestine, colon, rectum, and anal canal.

In fulfilling this function, the various components of bran pass through the intestinal tract virtually unchanged by the digestive process. Although they do not change chemically, the bran components do absorb and retain large quantities of moisture. The bran then acquires a jelly-like consistency, which, when mixed with food residue and body wastes, forms a soft yet bulky material. This consistency facilitates the movement of matter through the intestinal tract.

WHY BRAN IS THE BEST FIBER

Sources of fiber which possess the same moisture-retaining characteristics as bran can be found in a multitude of other foodstuffs, including vegetables, legumes, and fruits.

Bran is singled out for special attention due to its superiority over all other sources of fiber. Ounce for ounce, bran provides the quickest, most efficient, least expensive, and most beneficial results in attaining the proper functioning of the intestinal tract. This has proven true in repeated hospital applications, studies conducted among schoolchildren in many different countries, and controlled case studies of normal, healthy adults.[9,10,11,12,13]

Bran's superiority stems from the fact that the fiber of other foods such as vegetables, legumes, and fruits is partially digested. Consequently, less cereal-grain food (by volume) is required to attain satisfactory results, in comparison with other fiber-rich foods.

Whereas bran can restore bowel functioning to normal more quickly and safely than other alternatives, the consumption of other fiber-containing foods is *still* vital and necessary to good health.

HOW MUCH BRAN DO WE NEED?

Individual needs differ, according to body size and varying diets. If the patient prefers a diet devoid of the natural fiber found in grains, vegetables, legumes, and fruits, the amount of bran required to enable the stools to retain adequate moisture may be considerable. The bran might not improve the digestion of such food, but it could assist in its elimination.

For most people, attempting to alter poor eating habits overnight is unrealistic. For these individuals adding small amounts of unprocessed bran flakes to each meal can provide noticeable benefits in relieving symptoms of constipation. One to two teaspoons of bran should be taken *before* each meal.

Initially, one teaspoon of bran should be taken, gradually working up to two teaspoons at each meal. Few people can ingest bran by itself, as it is very dry and quickly soaks up the moisture in the mouth that facilitates swallowing.

Being tasteless to most people, bran can be added to milk, fruit juices, or water. It can also be readily added to sauces, soups, salads, gravies, and other moist foods.

When two rounded teaspoons of bran are taken with a small amount of water and then chewed, the bran is transformed into a soft elastic gel, similar to a piece of chewing gum. This indicates what occurs to the bran once it has entered the digestive system: It becomes a lubricant for the digesting foods.

Each individual should find the appropriate amount of bran for her or his digestive system by experimenting until the stools are moist yet bulky and can be easily passed.

ADDING BRAN TO THE DIET

There are a number of ways to add bran to the diet, the most effective being to add it to the food before it is served. This way everyone receives a minimum amount automatically, even the stubborn members of the family.

They will seldom notice that it has been added due to the ability of bran to take on the flavor of the foods to which it is added.

Those who require more bran can simply add more to their foods if the bran is placed on the table as a condiment. Few people realize that the bran of a wheat kernel contains more than half the vitamin B complex of the kernel. An ounce of bran has the vitamin B content of a large apple or five ounces of orange juice.[15]

It is suggested that a sugar bowl be filled with bran for the convenience of the members of the family and left on the table for all meals. This is, of course, in addition to adding bran in the process of cooking. Children enjoy shaking bran flakes from a large salt shaker or a commercial sugar container (restaurant size). Most large supermarkets carry these types of containers. A few packagers of unprocessed bran flakes even sell their product in such containers.

Refined Breakfast Cereals

Rather than purchase bran in its unprocessed form, some families might prefer to buy commonly advertised refined-bran breakfast cereals, many of which are heavily promoted as natural laxatives.

In order to get twelve to fifteen grams (or less than an ounce) of fiber per day, which is the suggested intake, the patient would have to consume prodigious amounts of these cereals. In a laboratory study of six well-known bran cereals, obtaining a sufficient amount of daily bran would require six servings in the case of two of the cereals, and almost half a box or more in the case of the other four.[16] If a patient's level of physical activity does not require such large amounts of cereal, it is far better to simply add a few teaspoons of unprocessed bran flakes to each meal.

LIMITATIONS OF BRAN

For Constipation

The consumption of bran is not an immediate answer to a bout of constipation. The reason for this is that the body requires a minimum of twenty-four hours to process bran once it has been ingested.

After Meals

Bran does not benefit the patient when it is consumed *after* a meal as much as it does *before* each meal. The mixing action of the stomach and intestines is more efficient when the bran is waiting in the stomach.

The bran may have to "catch up" with previously ingested food, thereby limiting its ability to add moisture to this food.

Poor Dietary Habits

Bran is not a substitute for a proper healthy diet. When refined products are consumed to the exclusion of fresh healthy foods, bran can only assist in reducing the frequency and severity of *stomachaches, constipation, and diarrhea.* It is far better for the patient to avoid digestive problems in the first place by consuming an intelligent balanced diet.

Iron Absorption

The seeds of wheat, corn, rice, soybeans, and peanuts contain large amounts of *phytic acid.* This compound reduces the absorption of iron in the small intestine.

Ascorbic acid, on the other hand is known to enhance the absorption of iron. In order to counterbalance the effects of phytic acid, the patient is advised to consume a healthy balanced diet—including an adequate amount of ascorbic acid. A glass of fresh orange juice daily, or a fresh orange is therefore recommended.[17]

Flatulence

This is the medical term for gas in the intestinal tract. When a good amount of beans, cabbage, peanuts, or bran is consumed, the patient may notice an excess amount of gas being passed shortly thereafter.

This is the main reason why bran should be slowly introduced into the digestive system. Starting with one teaspoon with each meal minimizes the initial flatulence. After the second or third week, the amount of gas passed quickly subsides. Fortunately, gas resulting from the consumption of unprocessed bran flakes is not particularly offensive.

Bran is a vital ingredient of any healthy diet, but it is not a substitute for:

1. a proper overall diet, and
2. timely, intelligent toilet habits.

Many patients attempt to use bran as a "neutralizer" after constipating foods or alcohol have been consumed to excess. Such efforts will be unsuccessful, because, as mentioned earlier, bran requires twenty-four hours to pass through the digestive system and thereby affect elimination. To be effective, bran must be consumed before or with meals on a *consistent* basis.

How much bran should be ingested daily depends mostly upon the amount of fiber-rich foods which are already being eaten. Initially, a patient should take one rounded teaspoon of bran before each meal, working up to two teaspoons over a period of two to three weeks. When the stools begin to pass smoothly without effort, the correct amount of bran is being consumed.

Chapter 8

A Better Diet

> "Digestive ailments lead all diseases in terms of time lost from work and money spent for hospitalization." [1]

ELEMENTARY HEALTH

In 1934 the American Book Company published an elementary school book entitled *Health in Good-Habit Land,* written by S. Weir Newmayer, A.M., M.D., and Edwin C. Broome, Ph.D., LL.D. The following excerpts from this book provide an excellent guide to a proper diet:

> "Good morning, Mary," said the grocer. His eyes twinkled when he smiled. "What can I do for you today?"
> "Please give me some oatmeal," said Mary.
> "Oatmeal?" asked the grocer.
> "Yes, sir," said Mary. "Mother says we need oatmeal to build up our bones and our muscles."
>
> Next they went to the baker's.
> "I should like some whole wheat bread," said Mary to the baker.
> "Why don't you buy white bread?" asked Billy.
> "Because white bread is not so good for us," answered Mary.

Mary stopped next at a vegetable stall.
The vegetable man asked, "What will you have?"
"I'll take a head of lettuce and two pounds of tomatoes for salad," said Mary. Then she bought spinach, beets, and potatoes.

"Now we shall get some fruit," said Mary.
"Come over here to the fruit stall with me."
They looked at the beautiful piles of oranges and apples.
Both looked so good she did not know which to take.
"I know," said Billy. "Get some of each."
And that is what she did.[2]

The foods which Mary is purchasing for her mother are almost precisely what we need in both the prevention and cure of hemorrhoids: whole-grain cereals, whole-grain breads, with fresh vegetables and fruits in abundance.

If the proper diet for good health was well-known more than forty years ago, we may wonder why more people do not consume a better diet? The answer to such a question, of course, varies with each individual. Many people prefer a food which is easily chewed and quickly swallowed, readily available, and sweet. Oftentimes, refined and sweetened foods meet these requirements better than unprocessed healthy foods. The media, via television, billboards, and magazines, generally promote the brand names of processed foods to the exclusion of unprocessed natural foods. How often do we see plain oatmeal, whole wheat bread, lettuce, tomatoes, potatoes, apples, or oranges advertised?

HEMORRHOID-DEVELOPING FOODS

A review of the types of foods and drinks which lead to the development of hemorrhoids may assist the patient in identifying problem areas.

White-Flour Products

The harmful effects of white-flour products can best be explained by describing the results of a comparative study with whole wheat bread by three British physicians:

> During the 1939–45 war, some of us participated in long-term balance studies in which we consumed, for several weeks, first 1 lb. of white bread daily, and later 1 lb. of whole wheat bread. Changes in bowel experience were considerable. On the white-bread regimen defaecation-times were irregular, and faeces were hard and were sometimes passed with pain.
>
> On the brown-bread regimen defaecation-times became regular and more frequent; the bulky stools were passed with neither strain nor discomfort. On the white-bread diet the urge to defaecate could be neglected, but much less so on the brown-bread diet.[3]

Sugar Products

Sugar is a very important subject in the discussion of hemorrhoids because it is so often substituted in various forms for the foods which should be consumed.

Sugar is a super-refined product. It has no fiber in its refined state. Nor vitamins. Nor protein. It requires no chewing at all. The greatest advantages of sugar to the manufacturer of refined foods are its relative cheapness and the ease with which it can be introduced into other foods. Once sugar has been fully refined, it can be turned into a liquid state which will mix readily with other processed foods.

Man has a natural sweet tooth and can digest reasonable amounts of natural sweeteners such as honey with no harmful effects. By introducing refined sugar into various processed foods, the food manufacturers take advantage of a natural human weakness in order to enhance the sale of their products.

Convenience Foods

These are food products in which the main advantages are their ease of preparation and rapid ingestion. They are frequently precooked or otherwise prepared for immediate sale or consumption. The fiber is often removed from such items by the processor so that the roughage will not clog the processing machines during manufacture. Fast-food outlets generally offer little in the way of nutritious foods. A milk shake made with artificial flavorings, artificial coloring, artificial sweeteners, emulsifying powders, preservatives for the ingredients, and powdered milk of unknown age has little room left for the nutritional items. Too many consumers care only about the taste of these items, a matter that is easily controlled by the addition of refined sugar.

Animal-Protein Foods

The nutritional value of most of these foods cannot be questioned when they are eaten in an unrefined, unprocessed state. The chief danger of these foods is that they are frequently consumed to the virtual exclusion of cereals, vegetables, legumes, fruits, and other fiber-containing foods. There is absolutely no fiber in meat, milk, cheese, eggs, yogurt, or other animal-protein products.

Medical authorities in the United States, Sweden, Norway, and Britain all suggest that adults should reduce fat in their diets to a level which is less than 35 percent of caloric intake.[4]

Recently, the Select Committee on Nutrition and Human Needs of the United States Senate stated that "Americans are eating far too many fatty foods and not enough carbohydrates." They also said that current eating habits:

> may be as profoundly damaging to the nation's health

> as the widespread contagious diseases of the early part of the century.[5]

Medical researchers in the United States have said that the "affluent diet" of this country is tied to six of the ten leading causes of death in the United States.[6]

Alcohol

We have already learned in Chapter 5 how the excess consumption of alcohol can cause hemorrhoids due to an enlarged liver. Alcohol also results in small dehydrated stools which cannot properly dilate the internal sphincter of the anal canal. This is why sufferers from third-degree hemorrhoids often experience some bleeding each time they over-indulge.

Hemorrhoid sufferers should significantly reduce their alcoholic intake, or simply omit this item from their menu. In any case, alcohol consumption should be limited to no more than a glass of beer daily or one cocktail per day.

RESULTING PROBLEMS OF THE REFINED DIET

The steady consumption of the aforementioned items results not only in a fiber-deficient diet but in a host of other problems.

Obesity (Overnutrition)

Consuming refined products and animal fats may also lead to what physicians term *overnutrition.* Researchers at the Worldwatch Institute in Washington, D.C., cite evidence that:

> victims of both undernutrition and overnutrition suffer a reduced life expectancy, are more susceptible to disease, and are less productive in their work.[7]

Obesity (overnutrition) is often called a disorder of people. This may be partially true in many cases, but more often it may be more accurately described as a disorder of diet.

Fiber-depleted products require far less volume in the stomach after ingestion, consequently requiring a greater amount of caloric intake before an individual becomes full. Unless the person leads a vigorous physical routine, this can cause the acquisition of undersirable excess weight.

Malnutrition

When meals are restricted to refined carbohydrates, such a diet can lead to severe protein and/or vitamin deficiencies. The individual may suffer from listlessness, slower physical activity, and reduced mental abilities.

In many of the emerging nations, great concern exists that the introduction of processed *baby foods* by multinational firms is leading to higher infant mortality rates and greater susceptibility to common diseases.

Abdominal Pain and Cramps

Abuse of the stomach is another by-product of the refined diet. When consumed to excess or in the wrong combinations, refined foodstuffs may overwork the stomach. The stomach is uniquely designed to handle most of these problems by simply regurgitating the food.

When regurgitation does not occur, much of the food may pass into the intestines and bloodstream, causing flu symptoms until the body has managed to rid itself of the poisons. How often we experience abdominal pain and cramps due to such products is difficult to measure. The evidence is soon gone or no longer in a recognizable form.

Not infrequently, errors in the manufacture of refined foods can result in harm to the consumer. In February, 1977, the Food and Drug Administration announced the recall of 19,000 cases of pretzels made by Pepperidge Farm, Inc. These pretzels had been sprinkled with *lye crystals* that could burn the tongues, mouths, and throats of purchasers. As it was revealed, lye and water were used to:

> give pretzels their glazed look. This process, properly carried out, is "safe" because pretzels absorb sodium hydroxide (lye) and the chemical is converted to sodium carbonate, a harmless substance, when pretzels are baked.
>
> In this case the sodium hydroxide apparently was not mixed properly. As a result, some of the chemical did not dissolve completely in the solution and subsequently got into the packages along with the pretzels.[8]

It is difficult to comprehend why a harmful chemical such as lye is permitted by the FDA to be utilized in the processing of a food solely for visual purposes.

MASTICATION OF FOOD

The proper chewing of food is important for three reasons. Digestive juices secreted in the mouth must mix with the food *before* it is swallowed. In the course of a day, the mouth may secrete as much as a quart of these digestive juices when food is properly masticated.[9]

Of course, the chewing must also reduce the size of the food particles to where they can readily be digested when they do reach the stomach.

A third vital function of chewing is to stimulate the secretion of the gastric juices of the stomach. Two quarts of gastric juices are normally secreted in one day. Without proper chewing, the food would receive insufficient digestive juices when it enters the mouth and gastric juices when it enters the stomach. This can also lead to abdominal pain and cramps.

Another indirect benefit of proper mastication is the prevention of overnutrition, or obesity. These juices fill the stomach just as food does, providing a sense of satiety before overconsumption can occur.

Since most of the fiber foods require considerable chewing, these foods are *good insurance* against overnutrition.

Luxury of Time

In this day and age, luxuries are becoming increasingly expensive and therefore prohibitive. One luxury which we can still have if we are willing to provide the time is the leisurely dinner. Make each meal a special time for relaxing. Savor every bite, chew the food until it can be easily swallowed, and wash it down with fresh juices or water. Enjoy meals with pleasant people.

The preparation of many fine meals depends more upon the choice of ingredients than hours of carefully overcooking perfectly good food in its fresh state. Food that is eaten fresh or briefly cooked contains more vitamins and more flavor than overcooked food.

THE FIBER FOODS

The following grains are listed in descending order by their ability to absorb and retain moisture. This ability is dependent upon the amount of indigestible fiber in each food.

Cereals

The following grains are listed in descending order by their percentage of crude fiber:

Millet, wholemeal	3 percent
Wheat, wholemeal	2
Rye, whole	2
Rice, brown	2
Millet, lightly processed	1.8
Corn, lightly milled	1.2
Oatmeal (unprocessed)	1.1
Oats, rolled	0.9
Rye, heavily milled	0.5
Rice, white unpolished	0.5
Rice, white polished	0.2

If ordinary white bread were included in this list,[10] it would bring up the rear at one-tenth of 1 percent.

Many people who try whole-grain breads, unprocessed oatmeal, and brown rice prefer it over the more easily chewed white breads, instant cereals, and white rice. The former foods are more "crunchy," tastier, and of course more satisfying than their refined counterparts. Whole-grain breads also provide other benefits—they do not get stuck to the roof of the mouth and do not fall apart around a hot dog or hamburger.

Whole-grain foods are also prime sources of Vitamin E, while other protein foods have little or no Vitamin E. This vitamin is believed to have an antioxidant feature which helps wash out decaying litter in the bloodstream.[11]

The only nationally advertised prepared breakfast cereals fit for consumption on the basis of the standards discussed in this chapter are shredded wheat and grape nuts. Both contain adequate fiber content in whole grains, with no sugar added. Bananas, peaches, strawberries, and other fresh fruit can be added for flavoring and additional fiber. The preceding chapter provides a discussion on the relative fiber content of many of the advertised bran cereals.

Legumes

Most legumes make excellent soups. They are also rich in protein content. Many societies which use legumes as their basic food source are free of most of the modern diseases discussed earlier.

Among generally consumed legumes, all having a high fiber content, are:

Lima beans
Soya beans
Kidney beans
Lentils
Chick peas

These foods also add a special touch to salads.

Nuts

The fiber content of nuts ranges between that of legumes and vegetables. Nuts are also frequently high in protein, such as in the case of almonds (40 percent). When snacks are necessary between widely spaced meals, nuts are an excellent offering both for children and adult guests.

Vegetables

These foods vary greatly in their ability to absorb moisture.

Carrots have the highest absorption rate of vegetables, a rate which is approximately one-half that of bran.

The following list shows the varying levels of moisture absorption in other vegetables, as they compare with carrots: [12]

Carrots	100 percent
Brussels sprouts	80
Eggplant	55
Cabbage, spring	55
Corn	55
Green beans	50
Lettuce	50
Cabbage, winter	50
Peas	50
Onions	44
Celery	44
Cucumbers	35
Tomato	30
Cauliflower	30
Potato	20
Turnip	18

Fruits

The fruits listed below are also compared with carrots in their ability to absorb moisture [13]:

Apple	85%
Orange	55
Pear	55
Banana	31

The amount of pulp in fruits determines the amount of fiber available. The *apple* is the superior fruit, just as the carrot is the superior vegetable. It is interesting to note that apple consumption in 1961 was seventy-five percent less than the figures for 1899.[14] This coincides in inverse proportion to the emergence of many diseases of the body caused by a lack of fiber content in the diet. Maybe there is something to the adage: "An apple a day keeps the doctor away."

Medical authorities often suggest that individuals who suffer from constipation should consume more liquids. By this, they do not mean more alcoholic or sugar drinks. Water is superior to these items in enabling the body to digest foods properly. Fruit juices are also better alternatives, particularly in their natural state.

Cereal grains and legumes are the best daily foods for fiber content. Fruits and vegetables are also good sources of fiber, but must be consumed in greater amounts than cereals and legumes in order to maintain good moisture content during digestion.

Unprocessed miller's bran should supplement the diet when fiber intake is believed to be too low. The amount of fiber one should consume is very easy to determine—it is the amount needed to pass stools of adequate bulk easily.

This bran is not a long-term substitute for whole grains though, as many medical researchers believe that whole-grain cereals are an important aid in keeping blood cholesterol levels in proper balance.[15] More research is required in the area of fiber and cholesterol levels at this time, but the indications are that most people benefit greatly by consuming fair amounts of whole grains.

Chapter 9

Toilet Habits

> "You people, complaining of your health, should pass large and bulky motions after every meal, and that to insure this, you should eat abundantly of whole meal bread, vegetables, and fruits."
>
> —*Hippocrates, 430 B.C.*

THE FIRST STEP

The consumption of a proper diet, as outlined in the preceding chapter, is the *most important part* of learning good toilet habits. It is useless to attempt the correction of poor toilet habits unless the diet provides "cooperating" stools.

NATURAL INSTINCT

When the body is prepared to eliminate waste, a specific signal is transmitted to the brain. This signal, called the *rectal reflex*, tells us that the rectum is full.

Young children often have the urge to go to the bathroom in the middle of, or immediately following, a meal. There is a good reason for this. It is not because they have "weak" bowels. It is because the entry of food into their stomach causes peristalsis to stimulate the movement of matter throughout the entire digestive tract. It is normal for peristalsis to cause body wastes to drop from the colon into the rectum. A child who asks to be excused from the dinner table to go to the bathroom is doing so because the body has properly given the signal that the rectum is full and requires emptying.[1] These children have not yet learned to suppress this natural instinct and thereby weaken their rectal reflex.

LEARNING BAD HABITS

The reasons why we postpone our bowel movements are quite numerous. Quite often it is because we have been taught to do so in childhood. When the parent insists that the child completes dinner before being excused to go to the bathroom, the child's rectal reflex is weakened. By the time dinner has been finished, this reflex may have entirely faded away. The next time the child experiences the urge for a bowel movement, the signal will be weaker. Eventually, when the rectal reflex has been ignored consistently, it may be difficult to distinguish when the reflex is occurring.[2]

Earlier in childhood when diapers are worn, the child automatically defecates when the rectal signal occurs. When the parent decides that the young child should be toilet trained, attempts are made to reverse the child's natural instinct. The child is set upon a potty and often required to remain sitting until a stool is produced. If the timing of the parent is ill-advised or the child has been fed constipating foods, this can be a very trying time for the child. Under such circumstances, the inevitable result is the development of the habit of straining while on the toilet. If the child is too young to understand fully the parent's demands, a certain degree of psychological damage may also occur.

Later, as adolescents, we're often in a hurry to do many other things than answer the needs of our body. During school we may be too embarrassed to request permission to be excused. After school we're too busy playing. It is easy to postpone the rectal reflex once the habit is established, since the rectum will send weaker signals the longer we make it our custom to inhibit the urge.

As Adults

The pressures of job and social requirements when we reach adulthood also tend to have a negative effect on our toilet habits.

In many jobs, especially those requiring early hours, it is not always convenient to give proper time to good nutrition and natural bowel functioning. Many persons have jobs which do not permit random breaks. Available breaks are prescheduled at specific times each day, which may or may not coincide with required bowel functioning.

Some jobs, especially in the military, simply do not allow for breaks at any time. Whether it be a soldier on a long hike or a pilot in a plane, natural bowel functioning must be totally ignored. Hemorrhoids are also considered to be quite common among pilots, possibly for this reason.

Social requirements have the same limiting effect on the ability of individuals to answer the rectal reflex. Rarely do visitors excuse themselves in another's home to have a bowel movement. Neither will the hosts do so until the visitors leave. When eating out at restaurants or banquets, people usually just ignore such needs.

Few people answer their natural urges away from their home or their job simply because they are not comfortable in unfamiliar surroundings at this time.

PLANNING BOWEL MOVEMENTS

Few people would seriously consider changing their jobs in order to permit an improvement in their bowel habits. A more realistic solution may be to alter eating habits.

It is a simple matter to accomplish this goal. First, a person must decide what time of the day is normally free for answering one's natural urges.

If the early morning (after waking) allows plenty of time, then the patient should plan the major meal of the day thirty-six hours prior to the early morning hours. This is the amount of time that our bodies require to digest and eliminate a healthy meal.[3] When we consume such a meal at 7 P.M. on a Monday evening, then the waste from that meal should be eliminated approximately thirty-six hours later, or early Wednesday morning.

NORMAL
36-HOUR ELIMINATION CYCLE

LARGEST MEAL OF DAY	CONSEQUENT BOWEL MOVEMENT	
MONDAY	TUESDAY	WEDNESDAY
MORNING →	NOON	
NOON →	EVE	
EVE →		MORNING

When an individual is badly constipated in the morning, it is not due to the previous evening. It is more likely due to his food intake thirty-six hours or more prior to his inability to have a regular bowel movement.

If *midday* is the first consistently available time for a bowel movement, then an attempt should be made to schedule the major meal in the early morning. Make breakfast the largest meal of the day. This will encourage the rectal reflex a day and a half later, at the noon hour. A secondary problem with this solution is that many people skip the noon-hour meal. Without food entering the stomach and stimulating peristalsis, there may not be a rectal reflex. If an individual wishes to have consistent bowel movements at midday, it will normally be necessary to consume a midday meal.

In the event that the early morning hours and the daylight hours both are rushed, then the heaviest meal should be the noon meal. When the midday meal is the major meal, normal elimination will occur thirty-six hours later or in the evening of the following day.

The necessity of consuming the diet suggested in the previous chapter cannot be overemphasized. The consumption of primarily refined foods in any form results in erratic bowel movements. Such foods vary in the amount of time they require to pass through our bodies. Some refined foods require only seventy-two hours, while others may take as long as five days.[4]

One must also be wary of refined products in supposedly healthy foods. Many restaurants, cafeterias, and even home cooks load salads, vegetables, and drinks with large quantities of sugar. The bread represented as whole wheat is often ordinary white bread with caramel coloring. Real whole wheat bread requires no coloring to have its brown appearance.

HOW OFTEN?

The answer to this question should be obvious by now: however often the body presents a genuine urge. If the body provides a signal, go to the bathroom and sit down on the toilet. This may be once, twice, or even three times a day.

Usually with a proper diet, there will be only one bowel movement per day. A few times a week, a second bowel movement per day is perfectly normal though. This type of regularity requires the patient to consume one *major* meal a day, at the *same time* each day. If all the meals are of a similar quantity, then the rectum may become full somewhat erratically.

Most people in the United States seem to consume their major meal in the evening. As a result their strongest rectal urge should occur in the early morning, thirty-six hours later. The peristalsis caused by a decent breakfast should initiate the bowel movement. A host of factors works against this natural functioning though. To restore regularity requires a study of many personal habits, job requirements, and various social pressures—not to mention diet.

The relief of having a good bowel movement at the same time each day may be just as rewarding to a general feeling of well-being as a good night's sleep.

THE URGE (THE RECTAL REFLEX)

When the rectal reflex occurs, one should immediately excuse oneself and head for the nearest bathroom or restroom.

After sitting down and relaxing, it is possible that the body will now fail to "produce." When this happens do not remain sitting on the toilet. Get up. Leave the bathroom and do not return again until another urge is experienced. Under such circumstances, many people will continue to sit and strain until they force a small bowel movement, or until it becomes obvious that there is really nothing to eliminate. This is wrong and probably contributes greatly to the development of the hemorrhoidal condition. People who are constipated and have made a habit of postponing their bowel movements tend to receive weaker rectal-reflex signals. These weak signals can be confusing and frustrating, causing much useless and harmful straining.

SITTING STYLE

Relaxing

Learning to *relax* completely at this time is of paramount importance. If a person has spent a good part of his/her life practicing the habit of straining on the toilet, it will take more than a few days to alter the habit.

After a few weeks of concentration and practice, one can expect some progress—provided the diet consists of healthy foods.

After sitting down, concentrate on something else besides straining. Reading is not recommended. Serious reading material may be one of the reasons partially responsible for previous lengthy sojourns in the bathroom.

Women who have experienced natural childbirth find that by counting and concentrating on something other than what they are undergoing, they are able to maintain an excellent state of relaxation. By using whatever methods seem best, one should also strive to maintain a relaxed state.

As one sits down, it should be in the same way one sits down at the dinner table or in the living room. Do not spread the buttocks. As a matter of fact, keep the buttocks a bit closer together than normal, as the design of the modern toilet seat naturally causes the buttocks to be spread excessively. By being careful to keep the buttocks closer together, one may be more able to maintain a relaxed state.

Experiment with various positions to determine which is the most comfortable. Positions may vary greatly as we are all of different sizes and shapes. It may help to use the arms somewhat for support.

It is also important that if clothes are worn they are not tight fitting, as this may inhibit the ability to relax. If necessary, disrobe entirely before sitting down.

Waiting

After being seated and then relaxing, *wait*. Wait for the bowel movement to begin of its own accord. As it begins, it may be helpful to brace a hand on the toilet seat in order to lift one buttock off the toilet seat. This assists in reducing straining. During the entire time one must *neither push nor strain* to assist in the elimination.[5]

Initially, an individual may not think much progress is being made to counterbalance the habit of straining. After a few weeks though, one should begin to notice that less straining is necessary. After a month or two, little or no straining may be noticed during bowel movements. Many people are amazed to discover that they can have a bowel movement without straining.

The body requires little conscious effort on our part to eliminate its waste material. We need only release the external sphincter muscle of the anal canal. If we disregard the requirements of the body for natural functioning, the body may gradually lose its ability to eliminate smoothly its wastes in the manner in which it is designed.

Required Time

When the bowels are functioning smoothly as a result of good dietary and toilet habits, it will rarely be necessary to remain seated longer than a minute.[6] In the majority of instances, it is even possible that the bowel movement will be completed fifteen seconds after it begins.

As soon as the bowel movement is completed, the patient should get off the toilet, cleanse the anal area, and leave the bathroom. Don't sit around to read the rest of the paper, or to see if you can muster a little bit more.

After elimination, with sufferers of prolapsing hemorrhoids there may be a continuing slight urge. The prolapsed hemorrhoid causes a sense of continuing fullness within the rectum. When *most* of the urge for a stool has been satisfied, one should get off the toilet quickly, tuck the hemorrhoid in again, and leave the bathroom. The patient may be surprised how often the continuing slight urge for a bowel movement disappears once the hemorrhoid is no longer protruding. Don't give the hemorrhoids the benefit of the doubt!

A state of constipation can also cause a continuing sense of fullness. In any case, do not remain sitting unless stools are being passed. To do otherwise simply encourages the development of larger hemorrhoids.

CLEANSING

Proper cleansing is another subject which receives rare attention in medical or other references.

The toilet paper, of course, should be *soft*. The modified anal skin which lines the outer two-thirds of the anal canal does not have the same resistance to abrasive materials as ordinary skin.

Another benefit of moistening toilet tissue is that the moist tissue picks up far more residue than dry tissue. When we clean our hands and other parts of our body, we don't use *dry* cloths or paper.

Replacement of Hemorrhoid

When a prolapsed hemorrhoid must be replaced, the toilet paper may have to come into contact with the distended lining of the inner third of the anal canal. This mucous membrane is particularly susceptible to abrasions and is frequently the source of anal bleeding related to hard stools and hemorrhoids.

Use of Moisture

The patient may have already discovered that the use of moisture on the toilet tissue facilitates the smooth replacement of prolapsed hemorrhoids. Water may be fully sufficient for such purposes, and when it is not available, one's own saliva is a good substitute. Saliva has a natural lubricating effect, in addition to always being available.

Commercial Lubricants

A number of commercially advertised lubricants for anal problems sometimes cause more problems than they solve.

When we wish to wash our bodies, we don't spread grease on our skin, especially if it is not water-soluble. Many of these commercial lubricants are difficult to remove readily, and the remaining residue may collect waste matter and other irritants. Itching in the anal area is often due to the lack of cleanliness, which these commercial lubricants tend to encourage. Mothers who have tried to clean their babies with these greases quickly learn not to do so.

URINATION

Do not postpone the need to urinate either. Urinate on demand, just as for defecation.

The urge to have a bowel movement can often be falsely signaled by an overfull bladder. After urination, the urge for a bowel movement sometimes disappears. When this occurs do not continue to sit on the toilet straining. Get off and leave the bathroom.

FLATUS

Passing gas from either end in mixed company can be embarrassing. Consequently, this particular bodily function is inhibited at an early age.

It should not be. It is a normal occurrence which permits the body to dispose of excess gases formed in the digestion and processing of food energy.[7] Of course, at the same time it should be said that discretion is appreciated by most people. If necessary, one can excuse oneself from company; use your imagination—there are many reasons why a person might move temporarily from one spot to another. It is certainly safer to move away than to "step on a frog."

Passing gas may or may not be a sign that a bowel movement is required. After passing the gas, wait to see if the urge to eliminate lessens. If it does not, one should certainly avail oneself of a bathroom and give the body an opportunity to find its own comfort.

TOILET SEAT DESIGN

There is little we can do when we are confronted with an uncomfortable toilet seat.

The design of the modern toilet seat is more conducive to reading than ease of elimination, which may explain the libraries in many bathrooms. In the Western world it has been supposed that the sitting position is the best for elimination. In less-developed societies (where hemorrhoids are virtually unknown), the Western-style toilet seat is quite rare.[8] These societies do very well in the squatting position.

Westerners may complain that the squatting position is uncomfortable. This is true, until one becomes accustomed to the position.

Unfortunately, this discussion is academic since facilities for squatting are simply not available in the Western world.

Persons with high blood pressure or other heart diseases should know that postponing bowel movements (and other poor habits discussed earlier) may result in constipation, which can lead to serious consequences in some cases.

A common complication of constipation among persons with heart disease is cardiac arrhythmia (irregularity in the rhythm of the heartbeat). It is estimated as the cause of one in twenty "natural" deaths and is more commonly referred to as "straining at stool." [9]

This straining consists of bearing down while holding one's breath, which "raises the blood pressure requiring more work to be done by the heart," according to Dr. Jesse Edwards, a cardiac pathologist at the University of Minnesota.[9] When the breath is finally expelled, Dr. Edwards states, "The blood pressure falls and may deprive the heart muscles of an adequate flow of blood." This upsetting of the heart rhythms can be fatal for persons who already have a heart problem—as in the case of Elvis Presley.

After the singer's death, an autopsy revealed:

> that strain had weakened and enlarged Presley's heart

> almost one-half beyond normal size and that the high-cholesterol foods Presley loved had left artery-narrowing deposits in his heart.[9]

Dr. George Nichopoulos, Elvis Presley's private physician, revealed that his patient had suffered from chronic constipation and further stated, "I felt it probably related to a long history of laxative abuse." [9]

REVIEW

1. To achieve regularity without straining, it may be necessary to change the diet (see Chapter 8).
2. Do not postpone bowel movements or the need to urinate. When the rectal reflex is ignored, it is weakened.
3. Adjust the timing of the largest daily meal so it precedes a regularly available time for bowel movements by thirty-six hours. This is the amount of time required to digest and eliminate a healthy meal.
4. Do not tarry on the toilet after the bowel movement is completed. Remove reading material from the bathroom. The time required to complete a bowel movement should seldom exceed one minute.
5. Permit the rectal muscles to expel the feces. The bowel movement should be accomplished with no conscious effort.
6. Before replacing a prolapsed hemorrhoid, moisten the toilet tissue with water or saliva. Moistened tissue also permits the anal area to be cleaned better.
7. When the major meal is in the evening, the patient should consume a decent breakfast, in order to initiate peristalsis, which then properly causes the rectal reflex.

Chapter 10

The Lack of Exercise

> "It is not the role of government to dictate life-style, but it is the proper role of government to educate our citizens and to aggressively stress the promotion of good health . . . the fact is, that if we were to improve our national eating, drinking, smoking, and exercise habits, we could be healthier, be happier, live longer, and save ourselves billions of dollars in the process."
>
> —*Jimmy Carter (October 1976)*

There is a relationship between the lack of exercise and the development of hemorrhoids. Lack of exercise, in combination with other bad habits, often leads to two conditions, both of which encourage hemorrhoidal formation: These are constipation and poor circulation.

CONSTIPATION

As this condition is believed to be the *major* cause of hemorrhoids, the lack of exercise can be considered an *indirect* cause of hemorrhoids to the extent that constipation is encouraged by inactivity.

In a discussion of the abuse of laxatives, the American Pharmaceutical Association suggests that often only a few nonmedical measures may be necessary for the treatment of constipation. These are:

1. a diet containing adequate roughage,
2. sufficient fluid intake,
3. *exercise*—if necessary, and
4. the establishment of proper stool habits.[1]

Medical references suggest frequent and moderate exercise for the prevention of many, if not most, serious disorders. Yet this simple expedient to better health is generally ignored by most people, who "don't have time" for such activities.

The Canadian Ministry of Health describes "excessive eating and smoking" as *"self-imposed risks* which are important underlying factors in each of the five major causes of death between age one and age 70." [2] The lack of exercise can also be described as a self-imposed risk.

Doctor Pruitt, author of one of the more recent medical texts (1938) on the subject of hemorrhoids, stresses several preventive measures, including:

1. a definite time of day for bowel movements,
2. a "moderate diet" including prunes, apples, potatoes, green vegetables and fruits,
3. the avoidance of highly seasoned foods and excessive alcoholic stimulants,
4. a sufficient amount of rest and exercise to maintain muscular tone, and
5. abstinence from the frequent use of drastic purgatives, such as calomel, rhubarb, and aloes . . .[3]

Doctor Pruitt also suggests that the use of any laxatives "should be discontinued as soon as constipation can be controlled by diet, regular habits, and *exercise*." [4]

POOR CIRCULATION

The body has developed a special unique system for controlling the anal canal which depends upon the rapid exit and entry of blood in the cavities of the anal cushions (see Chapter 2).

Physical activity is primarily responsible for the healthy return of blood to the heart through the veins. When the venal return of blood is poor, the reverse blood pressure from the liver back to the cavities of the anal cushions can be harmful to the tissue of the anal canal. This is of particular importance during bowel movements when the anal sphincters are open and relaxed.

Dr. Montague, author of *The Modern Treatment of Hemorrhoids,* tells us:

> Within our own times, we may observe that men accustomed to living a rough primeval life involving considerable muscular activity, as well as the subsistence on a coarse diet, are rarely troubled with this condition. Muscular action is efficient in preventing this condition in two ways:
>
> 1. by raising the physiological requirements for food so that overeating does not occur so readily; and, more important,
> 2. the fact that in a life of muscular activity there is no chance for portal plethora (engorgement of veins leading to the liver) or venous engorgement elsewhere in the body.[5]

The most frequent excuse given by persons who engage in little or no physical exercise is that their jobs do not permit the necessary free time, whether they are salaried or hourly wage earners, or housewives. For the workers with a problem, Dr. Pruitt makes the following suggestion:

> Change in occupation may be necessary when the patient leads a sedentary life or has irregular habits with little or no exercise.[6]

In addition, he states:

> Pregnant women should be warned to guard against constipation and advised to take liberal exercise and establish regular habits during the gestation period.[7]

When a change of occupation is out of the question, the patient will find that by rescheduling the major meal of the day, the timing of bowel movements can be easily controlled. How this is accomplished is fully described in each of the two preceding chapters.

Oversitting

Poor circulation due to inactivity is compounded by the position that most people assume when they are inactive. We sit at breakfast, while driving the car to work, while working, while at lunch, and again while driving home and then having dinner. The balance of the day may then be spent sitting in front of the television set.

Dr. Stanley DuBrin, a prominent physician in southern California, tells us:

> "The sitting person barely moves his legs and in such a sitting position he squeezes the hip and knee joints (and the blood vessels around them) hour after hour, day after day. Result: congestion of the lower extremities, damage to the liver cells, constipation due to digestive disturbances, hemorrhoids, varicose veins, cold legs and feet, edema, and leg ulcers." [8]

PLANNING EXERCISE

Having established the necessity of frequent, moderate exercise in order to remain healthy, careful consideration should be given to planning this activity.

Type of Exercise Needed

The first requirement is that the form of exercise be one which forces the blood to move more rapidly through the circulatory system. Such exercise need be no more vigorous than yoga to accomplish this goal. When the blood is pumping forcefully through the blood vessels, the patient should be well aware of the increased pulse.

The second requirement is that the exercise be one which is enjoyable. Exercise which is drudgery is soon postponed and discontinued.

If an individual really enjoys running alone over long distances, then this form of exercise may be appropriate.

Another form of exercise is one which requires the participation of a friend. The advantage is that company usually makes the exertion more enjoyable—even if the friend is a dog. Don't walk the dog; run it. The dog will certainly enjoy the outing more.

There are many sports which require little space, yet can be quite vigorous. Throwing two Frisbees simultaneously, two-person volleyball, Ping-Pong, racket ball, badminton—to name just a few.

Instead of driving everywhere, use a bicycle whenever possible. It may take a bit longer, but it is time well spent.

How Often?

The best answer to this question is: *daily*. Some benefits of exercise seem to last for only the following twenty-four hours, as this is as long as the blood remains well oxygenated.

A more realistic approach is to plan some form of vigorous exercise at least twice weekly. These exercises should also be evenly spaced during the week. Do not make the mistake of engaging in vigorous exercise only during the weekend and then doing nothing for the next five days. This is straining the body instead of properly exercising it.

If the weekend is the best time to get exercise, certainly use it, but a portion of a day in the middle of the week should also be set aside to keep the body well tuned.

Beginning Exercises

In planning any form of exercise, remember to begin such activity in *moderation*. To do otherwise is to invite the strain and pain of sore muscles. Permit the muscles to tone up slowly. Even yoga enthusiasts use a series of warm-up exercises before they attempt the more difficult positions.

Individuals who have led sedentary lives for many years may be well advised to seek a full physical examination prior to engaging in any form of major exertion. Many persons who have developed high blood pressure are totally unaware of their condition until they are notified by their physician during an examination. Even if an individual is still in the twenties, it may take months to regain the ability to throw a football or baseball over the same distance as in one's high school days.

The most important ingredient of any program should be that the activity is *fun*. When exertion can be enjoyed, it is much easier to sustain one's own interest, in addition to being easier to talk a friend into joining in the activity.

One's health is a precious thing, to be protected and cared for just as any other valuable possession. No amount of material possessions gained in working from dawn to dusk is worth the price of broken health.

Chapter 11

Suppositories and Ointments

Since advertising by the manufacturers of commercial suppositories and ointments appears to be directed toward relieving the symptoms of blood clots instead of hemorrhoids, it may be well to review again the nature of a blood clot.

Onset of a Blood Clot

When a fairly abrupt onset of pain occurs, accompanied by a swelling on the perimeter of the anus, a blood clot is the usual diagnosis. This swelling will be hard and tender to the touch.

Natural Resolution of a Blood Clot

Most victims of this affliction are initially unaware that the swelling and inflammation associated with a blood clot usually will diminish of their own accord. This spontaneous reduction of symptoms begins in most cases within forty-eight hours of the onset of pain.[1,2]

It is important that the reader have a thorough comprehension of the nature of a blood clot in order to understand why advertising of commercial hemorrhoid preparations is oriented toward the symptoms of a blood clot. For this reason, Chapter 4 should be reviewed prior to reading this chapter.

THE FEDERAL TRADE COMMISSION FINDINGS

Complaint

On August 28, 1964, the Federal Trade Commission caused a complaint to be filed alleging that American Home Products (the manufacturer of Preparation H) was guilty of making "false advertisements" implying "that the use of Preparation H Ointment and Suppositories" would:

1. Reduce or shrink piles;
2. Avoid the need for surgery as a treatment for piles;
3. Eliminate all itch due to or ascribed to piles;
4. Relieve all pain attributed to or caused by piles;
5. Heal, cure or remove piles, and cause piles to cease to be a problem.[3]

Qualifications of Witnesses

In the subsequent testimony before the Hearing Examiner, Walter R. Johnson, it is interesting to note the varying qualifications of the physicians appearing for the government versus the physicians who appeared for American Home Products.

The government called nine witnesess whose qualifications were described as follows:

> "Each specializes in proctology, which deals with diseases affecting the anus, rectum, and lower colon, including hemorrhoids. They are members of, and certified by, the American Board of Colon and Rectal Surgery, an exclusive group of less than 500 surgeons." [4]

These physicians were:

a. *Dr. Richard Hopping:* formerly Chief of Proctology,

Bethesda Naval Hospital, and presently President of the Medical Board and Chief of Proctologic Services, Saint Barnabas Medical Center, Newark, New Jersey; author of a number of articles on disorders of the anus, rectum and lower colon.

b. *Dr. Sylvan Manheim:* formerly chief of the Rectal Clinic, Mount Sinai Hospital, New York, New York and Clinical Professor of Surgery for Rectal Diseases, New York Medical College; presently Consulting Proctologist, Mount Sinai Hospital. Author of the book *Proctology,* published by Oxford University Press in 1943; co-author of a number of articles in the field.
c. *Dr. W. Martin Marino:* Chief, Department of Surgery, Division of General Surgery, Division of Proctology, The Brooklyn-Cumberland Medical Center.
d. *Dr. Samuel W. Eisenberg:* Clinical Professor of Proctology, Temple University Medical Center.
e. *Dr. Joseph B. Sarner:* Senior Attending Proctologist, Einstein Medical Center, Philadelphia; instructor in proctology at Graduate School of Medicine, University of Pennsylvania.
f. *Dr. Andrew J. McAdams:* Chief of Department of Proctology, Division of Surgery, Western Pennsylvania Hospital.
g. *Dr. Karl Zimmerman:* formerly President of the American Proctologic Society, author of over 30 articles and papers in the field.
h. *Dr. Charles Evans Pope:* Head of the Proctologic Department, St. Francis Hospital, Evanston, Illinois; author of 30 papers and articles in the field.
i. *Dr. Durand Smith:* Chief of the Surgical Rectal-Proctoscopy Clinic at Northwestern University Medical School.[5]

Although American Home Products called more witnesses than the government during the hearing, only one was experienced as a proctologist. This was Dr. William Lieberman of Brooklyn, New York, at the time Director of the Department of Proctology, Unity Hospital, Brooklyn, New York.[6]

Defining a Blood Clot

The findings of the Commission provide the following description of a blood clot:

> An "external thrombotic hemorrhoid" is a blood clot under the surface of the skin located in the immediate vicinity of the anal opening . . . It is also referred to as an "anal hematoma" or a "perianal thrombosis." [7]

Natural Resolution

During the testimony before the Hearing Examiner, it was noted that: "The discomforts and symptoms of hemorrhoids (*Author's Note: more correctly "blood clots"*) frequently subside spontaneously." [8] The following remarks concerning blood clots were made by the proctologists in attendance:

> *Dr. Hopping:* "Nature and the resources of the body frequently take care of the immediate acute situation and heal it in the course of time. They don't heal the hemorrhoids."
>
> *Dr. Marino:* "The swelling subsides. Any infection or inflammation that may be present subsides. Irritative bowel movements may be relieved, and this would effect some degree of relief of an acute process, an acute hemorrhoidal situation."
>
> *Dr. Eisenberg:* "Just mother nature and time, both of which are excellent helpers, and we see patients many times who are made appointments for an acute episode of what they call hemorrhoids and if we are not able to see them for several days, by the time they come in, much of their symptomatology has been relieved, spontaneously, though they have done nothing. So we know

> from experience that many of these complications will subside spontaneously."
>
> *Dr. McAdams:* "The inflammatory reaction around the hemorrhoids was induced perhaps by constipation or diarrhea or excessive lifting or straining. It subsides in the course of that which makes life possible for all of us, Mother Nature's tendency to correct abnormalities. Time is a great healer."
>
> *Dr. Zimmerman:* "Well, if a person has irritation in the hemorrhoidal area and the irritation subsides, just like irritation on the hand, the leg, or anywhere else, if it subsides spontaneously, the body healing will take care of it and the patient will gradually become free from symptoms even though nothing is done."
>
> *Dr. Pope:* "Time itself plays its biggest factor as far as treatment other than surgery and other than injection treatment. Topical application of heat may help and benefit. After a period of time, nature herself causes the subsidence of whatever symptoms are present." [9]

The opinion of these proctologists is that blood clots (often misidentified as hemorrhoids) subside in severity *of their own accord,* regardless of the application of commercial products.

OPINION OF THE "GOVERNMENT" PROCTOLOGISTS

In summarizing the testimony of the nine proctologists who were witnesses for the government, the Hearing Examiner stated:

> Based upon their education, training, and experience, the nine proctologists gave opinion testimony, the substance of which was that Preparation H Ointment and Suppositories containing the ingredients listed in the formula, when used as directed, will not:
>
> 1. Reduce or shink piles;

2. Avoid the need for surgery as a treatment for piles;
3. Stop all itch due to piles;
4. Relieve all pain due to piles;
5. Heal, cure or remove piles or eliminate the problem of piles; and
6. Have any therapeutic effect upon piles or the symptoms thereof in excess of affording temporary relief of minor pain or minor itching associated with piles.[10]

The basic reason why commercial suppositories and ointments have no overall beneficial effect on hemorrhoids is succinctly stated by Dr. Zimmerman:

> the hemorrhoids are varicose veins, they are under the skin or under the membrane, and whatever is put on top of the skin or membrane can have little effect on what is under it.[11]

OPINION OF THE FEDERAL TRADE COMMISSION

The following opinion of the Federal Trade Commission was rendered on December 16, 1966. It ordered American Home Products to:

> cease and desist from disseminating or causing the dissemination of any advertisement . . . in connection with the offering for sale . . . of Preparation H Ointment or Suppositories . . . which:
>
> 1. Represents directly or by implication that the use of such product will:
>   a. Reduce or shrink hemorrhoids or hemorrhoidal tissue or membranes or reduce or shrink swelling associated with hemorrhoids;
>   b. Avoid the need for surgery as a treatment for hemorrhoids or hemorrhoidal symptoms;
>   c. Heal, cure or remove hemorrhoids or eliminate the problem of hemorrhoids;
>   d. Afford any relief from pain or itching attributed to or caused by hemorrhoids in excess of affording

some temporary relief in some cases of pain and itching associated with some types of hemorrhoids;

e. Afford any other type of relief or have any other therapeutic effect upon the condition known as hemorrhoids or upon any of the symptoms or manifestations thereof.[12]

MODIFICATIONS OF FTC ORDER

Unfortunately, the Federal Trade Commission later modified this order (1969 and 1970) in response to direction from the U.S. Court of Appeals (Sixth District). According to the record of proceedings of the FTC, both the members of the Commission and the Court of Appeals failed to understand or to distinguish the difference between a hemorrhoid and a blood clot.[13,14,15,16,17] Due to this misunderstanding, we now see and hear much of the same claims in television, radio, newspaper, and magazine advertising to which we were exposed prior to 1966.

OPINION OF THE EDITORS OF *CONSUMER REPORTS*

In *The Medicine Show,* a medical book written for the lay person and published by the editors of *Consumer Reports* in 1974, the following opinions are given:

> Suppositories, although widely advertised, are of little proven value for either internal or external hemorrhoids. Nor do suppositories have any beneficial effect on the pain of hemorrhoids.[18]

OPINION OF THE AMERICAN PHARMACEUTICAL ASSOCIATION

The 1973 edition of the *Handbook of Non-Prescription Drugs* (published by the American Pharmaceutical Association) reveals:

> the patient frequently seeks self-medication and is undoubtedly influenced to a great degree by the unsupported advertising claims that some manufacturers make for the preparations they recommend for the treatment of this affliction. Literally scores of preparations are available. Some of the products require a prescription but a great number are sold over the counter. Undue reliance on these preparations and failure to seek medical advice may have serious consequences.[19]

The "serious consequences" alluded to in the above statement include many ailments whose symptoms are similar to those of hemorrhoids, such as:

1. an anal fissure,
2. cryptitis (inflammation of the anal valves),
3. a fistula (chronic lesion or cavity in the neighborhood of the anus),
4. a benign tumor of the lower colon,
5. an abscess,
6. a malignant cancer of the rectum.[19]

There are many other serious disorders which occur higher up in the intestinal tract that can cause symptoms thought to be due to hemorrhoids. When the patient seeks self-medication instead of proper medical attention, these disorders may be permitted to progress to the point where considerable suffering may result.

The use of commercial preparations is a poor substitute for an intelligent diet and improved toilet habits.

Whereas an improvement in personal habits and proper medical attention can halt the further development of hemorrhoids, there is little doubt that commercial products provide only *temporary* relief of some minor symptoms.

Chapter 12

Laxatives

That the abuse of laxatives should lead to the very condition which they are advertised to remedy is ironic but true.

We are told in the *Handbook of Non-Prescription Drugs* (1973) that:

> Chronic constipation, not of organic origin is most often the result of the unnecessarily prolonged use of irritating or mineral oil laxatives.[1]

Dr. Louis A. Buie, Sr., author of *Practical Proctology* (1960), states that:

> Hemorrhoids rarely afflict youths, but constipation frequently begins during adolescence. The use of laxative agents probably plays a significant role. Many persons begin the use of such agents while in their teens. By the time they become adults, many persons cannot remember when they could maintain themselves without a laxative agent, and some cannot remember when they had a normal bowel movement.[2]

The editors of *Consumer Reports* tell us:

> The misuse of laxatives is another important cause of chronic constipation. Moreover, there are comparatively few users of cathartics (laxatives) who have not suffered from fissure of the anus or hemorrhoids. If you think

> you have chronic constipation, the first thing to do is stop taking laxatives.[3]

Dr. Pruitt, author of *Hemorrhoids* (1938), reveals:

> Drastic cathartics and other drugs . . . produce congestion of the pelvic veins and tend to increase peristalsis and distention of the hemorrhoidal plexus.[4]

Dr. Montague, in *The Modern Treatment of Hemorrhoids* (1925), tells us:

> One of the most flagrant, if not the most frequent, exciting causes of hemorrhoidal formation is the abuse of cathartics.[5]

SEEK MEDICAL ADVICE FIRST

The advice provided in medical references not only stresses the dangers of the overuse of laxatives, but repeatedly suggests that the victim of constipation should use laxatives only upon the advice of a physician.

Fifty years ago Dr. Montague, in discussing the abuse of laxatives, stated:

> This group of medicines are legitimate therapeutic agents only when definitely indicated, and a physician is the best judge of that.[6]

More recently, we are told in an official publication of the American Pharmaceutical Association that:

> There is no class of nonprescription drugs in which professional guidance is needed more than it is with the use of laxatives.[7]

Medical consultants to Consumer's Union suggest:

> that you avoid any laxatives containing chemicals that act as bowel stimulants, unless advised by your physician.[8]

It is doubtful that many people heed this advice, as the sale of more than 700 proprietary laxative preparations totaled more than $192 million as recently as 1969.[9]

In the opinion of the editors of *Consumer Reports:*

> There is no doubt that laxatives have contributed more to the ills and discomforts of mankind than the condition they are supposed to relieve.[10]

ABUSE AND HARMFUL SIDE EFFECTS

Ignoring Serious Illnesses

The greatest danger in relying on these self-medications is that a *serious* disorder may either be ignored or even further aggravated by the ingestion of laxatives.

Many people incorrectly believe that abdominal pain is a symptom of constipation. The medical consultants to Consumer's Union tell us:

> Instances of a ruptured appendix with peritonitis have been recorded in patients who assumed their abdominal pain was caused by constipation and so dosed themselves with laxatives. Constipation is rarely associated with severe abdominal pain. Nor does the presence of pain mean the bowels need to be cleaned out.[11]

Diverticulitis and cancer of the rectum may also cause constipation. Both require *prompt medical attention.*

Mineral Oil

Mineral oil is one of the most frequent ingredients in laxatives. The dangers associated with its frequent ingestion cannot be overstressed. They include:

1. chronic constipation,[12]
2. incompetence of the ileocecal sphincter (this sphincter's function is to prevent backflow of fecal content from the colon into the small intestine),[13]

3. rectal leakage and resulting irritation,[14]
4. interference with absorption of nutrients (vitamins A, D, and E),[15]
5. retardation of gastric emptying time, especially when taken just before a meal,[16] and
6. lipid pneumonia, a condition in which mineral oil has coated the pharynx, thereby gaining access to the trachea and then the lungs.[17]

Anthraquinone Laxatives

These include cascara sagrada, senna, rhubarb, aloe, and their derivatives. "Their main side effects are *excessive* catharsis (evacuation of the bowels)," according to the *Handbook of Non-Prescription Drugs* (1973).[18] The same source reveals that the active principles of these substances "appear in body secretions and during lactation they may be present in the milk in sufficient concentrations to affect nursing infants."

Phenolphthalein

The major hazard of this ingredient is "usually electrolyte and fluid deficits resulting from excessive catharsis."[19] In addition:

> In susceptible persons a large dose may cause diarrhea, colic, or cardiac and respiratory distress and even collapse. The second type of reaction is dermatitis. The rash is polychromatic and ranges in color from pink to deep purple.[20]

Oxyphenisatin and Acetate

The properties of these substances resemble those of phenolphthalein. Recent reports have revealed:

> toxicities attributed to this compound when it is used for prolonged periods.

One report concerned four women, ages 47 to 86 years, who had a similar, moderately severe illness characterized by fatigue, vague abdominal symptoms, jaundice and moderate hepatomegaly (a liver disorder).

When the use of the laxative was discontinued, the symptoms and serum abnormalities were improved. Resumption of the laxative caused the return of jaundice in a period of from two days to six weeks.[21]

Bisacodyl

The side effects of this substance are less severe than many others, being "abdominal pains (cramps), nausea, and dizziness."[22] In its suppository form, it may produce a burning sensation in some individuals.[23]

Calomel

This laxative substance results in greenish stools, which is not harmful. Problems may arise with this ingredient if it is retained too long in the intestinal tract:

> If for any reason the elimination of the drug is retarded, appreciable amounts of the toxic mercuric ion can be absorbed. In such cases a saline laxative is indicated for removal of the drug from the intestinal tract.[24]

Saline (Salt) Laxatives

These laxatives remove water from the stomach to the small intestine, therefore they "should be administered with enough water to ensure protection from loss of water."[25] Further:

> Cathartics containing the sodium ion may be toxic to those who suffer from edema and congestive heart disease. Dehydration may occur from the repeated use of hypertonic solutions of saline cathartics and such a re-

sult can be exhausting to those who cannot afford fluid loss.[26]

Bulk-Forming Laxatives

These laxatives should not be taken in dry form, as "esophageal obstruction has occurred when they have been swallowed dry." They may also cause "fecal impaction or intestinal obstruction" when taken "by persons with intestinal ulcerations, stenosis or disabling adhesions." [27]

Other Laxatives

There are many, many more substances commonly used in commercially advertised laxative products which have questionable side effects on the user. Perhaps a description of the "perfect" laxative by the *Handbook of Non-Prescription Drugs* (1973) will provide some guidance to the reader:

> An ideal laxative should be nonirritating and nontoxic and should act only on the descending and sigmoid colon. Within a few hours it should produce one normally formed stool. Its action should than cease and permit the resumption of normal bowel activity. Such a laxative is not now available.[28]

ALTERNATIVES

The preceding chapters on bran, diet, toilet habits, and exercise offer the victim of frequent constipation more than adequate instruction in the treatment of the disorder. These remedies are all directed at the most frequent causes of constipation.

When these measures do not alleviate the condition within a week, medical advice should be promptly sought.[29]

Any laxative which is ingested should be by direction of a physician only, after proper discussion of one's symptoms.

When the patient feels compelled to use a self-remedy for constipation, perhaps the best advice is contained in *The Medicine Show* (1974):

> Some people may find it more natural, if not as convenient, to use an enema instead of a laxative. As authorities have been saying for many years, it does seem unreasonable to upset 25 feet of intestine with a cathartic when the trouble is in the last 8 inches—the rectum and anal canal. An enema consisting of a pint of tepid tap water is generally sufficient.[30]

Chapter 13

Enemas

Although enemas are considered generally superior to laxatives in relieving constipation and cleansing the bowels, frequent use can also lead to serious side effects. For this reason, whenever they are utilized it should be with *caution* and preferably after consulting a physician.

FLUID OR SUPPOSITORY FORM?

There are two basic forms of enemas, the commonly used *fluid* type and another form, which is gaining increasing acceptance—the *suppository* enema.

The insertion of a suppository enema requires far less time than a fluid one, in addition to being a more aesthetically acceptable method for the patient.

A four-month study at the Mayo Clinic of the comparative cleansing efficiency of the two revealed that the suppository method provided excellent results 80.7 percent of the time; whereas, the fluid enema provided similar results 77.4 percent of the time.[1]

Since the suppository enema appears to yield excellent results and is much easier to administer, it may soon become the preferred method both in hospitals and at home.[2]

SUPPOSITORY ENEMAS

There are several different types of suppository enemas, including glycerin, bisacodyl, senna concentrate, and carbon dioxide-releasing chemical agents.

Glycerin suppositories have been used for many years in the relief of constipation or "supposed" constipation in both adults and infants. They should be used cautiously as:

> Their occasional use does no harm, but most physicians believe that for many individuals frequent use can cause irritation of the anus and mucous membrane of the rectum.[3]

The more recently developed bisacodyl and carbon dioxide suppositories have been found to be "quite adequate" in the preparation for examination by a proctologist.[4] They are also promoted for use in postoperative, antepartum (prenatal), and postpartum care.

The *Handbook of Non-Prescription Drugs* (1973) states:

> Recent reports of clinical investigations of the carbon dioxide releasing type of suppository suggest, however, that it might serve as a beneficial replacement for some of the uses of the enema.[5]

The major drawback of the frequent use of suppository enemas is the same as that for fluid enemas:

> too frequent enemas—even once a week, for some people—can result in inability to initiate a bowel movement without recourse to an enema.[6]

FLUID ENEMAS

There are a great variety of fluids commonly used for enemas, including water, normal saline (salt) solutions, hypertonic saline solutions, milk, vegetable oils, soapsuds, hydrogen peroxide, and other commercial solutions.

Result of Frequent Usage

Problems arising from the "injudicious use" of these fluids are numerous and varied:

> Enema fluids containing substances foreign to the bowel have caused mucosal changes or spasm of the intestinal wall. Hydrogen peroxide enemas have caused proctitis and even gross hemorrhage. The mucosal irritation has been of sufficient extent to resemble the early changes of ulcerative colitis. Water intoxication has resulted from the use of tap-water or soapsuds enemas in the presence of megacolon.[7]

When in doubt as to which fluid to use, the patient is advised to use plain water. The medical consultants to Consumer's Union advise:

> An enema consisting of a pint of tepid water is generally sufficient.[8]

When patients are preparing for an examination, the *Handbook of Non-Prescription Drugs* (1973) states:

> they are usually directed by the physician to use a tap-water enema until they get clear returns.[9]

Administration of the Fluid Enema

After the possibility of serious illness has been eliminated, the patient should exercise great care in self-administering a fluid enema.

The amount of fluid used should vary with the purpose of the enema. If the only purpose is to relieve constipation, then only one pint should be necessary. When the patient is preparing for an examination, then three pints of fluid may be needed to obtain clear returns (water free of fecal content). The fluid should be slightly warm or near room temperature.

The patient should be in a horizontal position, with the buttocks in an elevated position, as gravity is necessary to properly distribute the fluid. A semikneeling position may work best.

The nozzle of the container should be adequately lubricated, and when a second enema is needed, the nozzle should be lubricated again. The tip of the nozzle should be directed toward the navel and should be inserted very slowly, never forcibly. The anal sphincter muscles should be permitted to relax before and during insertion.

After the nozzle is properly inserted, the container should be gently squeezed until empty or until the rectum is full.

The fluid should be retained until lower abdominal cramping is felt. This may vary from somewhat less than a minute to five or ten minutes. The patient should not strain in order to eliminate the fluid.

As mentioned earlier, "clear returns" means the passage of fluid which is free of fecal matter. Many persons exhaust themselves in an attempt to pass perfectly clear water, which is not necessary.

Professional advice is suggested in the use of any substance which is to be inserted into the rectal area.

Neither fluid nor suppository enemas should be used regularly.

Suppository enemas, having an effectiveness similar to that of fluid enemas, may be preferred due to their ease of application.

The patient should remember that the use of an enema will not affect the cause of the problem. It will not treat constipation effectively when constipation persists. This is better accomplished by seeking medical attention and giving consideration to those personal habits which may be contributing to the state of constipation.

Chapter 14

A Natural Cure

There is no pill that cures hemorrhoids, no medicinal fluid, no suppository, no ointment, and no powder. Modern pharmacology and medicine have not yet developed an over-the-counter or prescription drug in any form that cures hemorrhoids, and it is doubtful that they ever will.

There are many drugs now on the market which are represented as beneficial to hemorrhoids. The use of most of these commercially advertised products simply permits the real causes of the hemorrhoids to remain untreated. When these causes are ignored, hemorrhoidal development is thereby encouraged.

Many individuals are convinced that the "answers" to an illness or a disorder of the body must be attractively packaged and have a price tag on it to be of any worth. For these persons there may be no natural cure. It is not possible to package better toilet habits, an improved diet, the will power to exercise, or the intelligence to avoid laxatives and other potentially harmful products.

CHANGING HABITS

Although none of the foregoing measures need involve additional expense (some may even mean a savings), they may require an altering of long-established habits.

For those persons who consider an improvement of poor habits to be "too high a price," the best answer to their problems may be found in the last chapter of this book. Hopefully, hemorrhoids will be the worst digestive or elimination disorder they will encounter.

For others who are more conscious of their overall health, it is quite possible to cure first-, second-, and *some* third-degree hemorrhoids.[1,2,3,4,5] Where a cure is no longer possible due to the quantity of prolapsing tissue, at least the further development of a hemorrhoidal condition may be halted. To obtain optimum results does require the serious and permanent improvement of many personal habits affecting the digestive and elimination systems. The hemorrhoid sufferer cannot "pick and choose" among those areas that need improvement. To ignore one's toilet habits while upgrading the diet will be fruitless, and vice versa.

As Shakespeare tells us: "The eye seeth not itself." If you have developed a serious hemorrhoidal complaint and feel that your personal habits could not be responsible, then maybe you should ask close friends and family members what they think of any of those personal habits which may be related to hemorrhoid growth.

Having a color TV in the bathroom does not encourage good toilet habits. Fast-food outlets are not good sources of fresh unadulterated foods. Standing on one's feet during the working day does not constitute exercise.

The speed with which personal habits can be improved will determine the amount of time required to reverse or halt the growth of hemorrhoidal tissue. Results may be realized in a few days, but more often a number of weeks or months may be required. Toilet habits are not as easily altered as a menu and may require some practice before they are perfected.

The *most important* step for all individuals who believe that they suffer from hemorrhoids is to ascertain the degree of hemorrhoidal development. This can be determined best with an examination by a proctologist.

The problem may not even be hemorrhoids; instead it may be one of numerous other difficulties often confused with hemorrhoids. In the words of Dr. Montague:

> They are, however, not as frequently present as they are diagnosed.[6]

PART III

Medical Treatment

Chapter 15

Finding the Cryosurgeon

Although cryotherapy in the treatment of hemorrhoids has been practiced since 1968, it is still a relatively new medical procedure. Consequently, finding a cryosurgeon within the specialty of proctology may require some looking. Ten years ago expectant parents had to make a similar search for obstetricians well versed in the technique of "natural childbirth." Hopefully, cryosurgeons in proctology will eventually become as readily available as such obstetricians now are.

In the search for a cryosurgeon, one should always begin by asking for a proctologist. To simply ask for a cryosurgeon without specifying the specialty may be confusing, as cryotherapy is used to treat many disorders besides those of the lower intestinal tract.

There are a number of different approaches to locating a cryosurgeon.

SCHOOLS OF MEDICINE

This is a good place to start, since many schools of medicine are quite interested in developing more effective and acceptable methods of delivering medical care. When contacting a school of medicine, one should ask first for either the Department of Surgery or the Department of Proctology. After establishing contact with a proctologist, an inquiry can be made concerning the available methods of treatment.

When the school of medicine does not offer this form of treatment, it may be able to refer the patient to another source of medical care which does practice cryotherapy.

LOCAL HOSPITALS

When contacting a hospital, do not expect the receptionist or all members of the hospital administration to be able to answer questions concerning cryotherapy. Such persons can be totally unfamiliar with the term, especially as it applies to the treatment of hemorrhoids. This may be due to the fact that most cryotherapies are performed in a physician's office, not in a hospital.

With a hospital one should first ask for the Department of Proctology. After the offices of the chief proctologist have been contacted, an inquiry concerning the use of cryotherapy can be made.

Just as in the case of a school of medicine, due consideration should be given to the limited amount of time that these proctologists have available to counsel potential patients. When these specialists cannot offer the freezing procedure at their own institutions, they are often in a good position to know of others that do.

MEDICAL SOCIETIES

Calling the local medical society should only be a last resort. Normally it is useless to ask the medical society for the names of proctologists who practice cryosurgery. It's also difficult to obtain the names of more than three proctologists per phone call.

It may be necessary to spend several days calling various proctologists until one is found who can serve your interests. On occasion, the reactions of a few physicians' offices which offer only those methods of treatment which were available 2000 years ago may prove interesting. It is amazing how long new medical procedures can take to become well known, aside from being widely practiced.

When local schools of medicine, hospitals, and medical societies cannot provide assistance, it may be necessary to travel to a larger city in order to find a proctologist trained in cryotherapy.

GOING TO THE SOURCES

When writing to a distant cryosurgeon, a short note with an enclosed self-addressed, stamped postcard might be the best means of communication.

When a telephone call is made to the office of a cryosurgeon, one should be considerate of his available time. Should the physician be busy, leave a message concerning the nature of the call and offer to call back later. By contacting a proctologist in New York State whose name had appeared in *The Wall Street Journal*, I was able to locate quickly a cryosurgeon in southern California.

The following list provides the names of physicians who perform cryotherapy as well as medical institutions where such treatment of hemorrhoids is available.

The East:

Robert Ehrlich, M.D., Center Professional Building, 280 Washington St., Suite 208, Brighton, Mass. 02135.

Sanford Savin, M.D., 2660 Main St., Bridgeport, Conn. 06606.
also: Chief of Proctology, Park City Hospital.

Harold T. Klein, M.D., D.I.B.P., 33 Forest Avenue, Stamford, Conn. 06902.

James P. Fleming, M.D., 125 Meigs St., Rochester, N.Y. 14607.
also: Chief, Department of Colon and Rectal Surgery, Park Ridge Hospital.

Edwin Alford, M.D., 50 High St., Buffalo, N.Y. 14203.
also: Professor of Colon and Rectal Surgery, General Hospital, University of Buffalo.

Arthur A. Rand, M.D., Parker Towers, 104–60 Queens Blvd., Forest Hills, N.Y. 11375.
also: Assistant Clinical Professor of Surgery, Albert Einstein College of Medicine, New York City.

Frederic C. Singer, M.D., 26 Hamilton Ave., Yonkers, N.Y. 10705.
also: Chief of Proctology, Yonkers Professional Hospital.

Changyul Oh, M.D., 1212 Fifth Ave., New York, N.Y. 10029.
also: Chief of Rectal Service, Mt. Sinai School of Medicine, City University of New York.

Irving G. Larkey, M.D., 119 Clinton Ave., Irvington, N.J. 07111.

Harold Solomon, M.D., 40 Union Ave., Irvington, N.J. 07111.

R. Douglas Cassel, M.D., 2405 Linglestown Rd., Harrisburg, Pa. 17110.
also: Clinical Instructor, Hershey Medical Center, Pennsylvania State University, Hershey, Pa.

Richard G. Ulrich, M.D., 2405 Linglestown Rd., Harrisburg, Pa. 17110.
also: Clinical Instructor, Hershey Medical Center, Pennsylvania State University, Hershey, Pa.

John O'Connor, M.D., 916 19th St., N.W., Washington, D.C. 20006.
also: Department of Surgery, Georgetown University, Washington, D.C.

Stanley P. Wegryn, M.D., Director, Louis S. Wegryn Memorial Clinic, 4301 Sanibel-Captiva Rd., Sanibel Island, Fla. 33957.

Mid-America:

A. Gerson Carmel, M.D., 1267 Hicks Blvd., Fairfield, Ohio 45014.

S. K. Kim, M.D., The Hartford Clinic, S.C., 1113 East Sumner St., Hartford, Wisc. 53027.

James R. Weber, M.D. Weber Medical Clinic, 1110 West Main St., Jacksonville, Ark. 72076.

Bert Myers, M.D., School of Medicine, Louisiana State University, New Orleans, La. 70112.

The West:

Paul E. McGuff, M.D., 2909 Hillcroft, Houston, Tex. 77057.

J. J. Bernhard, D.O., Paradise Valley Medical Center, 13402 N. 32nd St., Phoenix, Ariz. 85032.

A. M. Ahmed, M.D., 1300 No. Vermont Ave., Suite 409, Los Angeles, Calif. 90027.

Martin I. Lewis, M.D., Director, Airport Medical Clinic, 2192 Martin St., Irvine, Calif. 92715.

Thomas N. Poore, M.D., 2920 Broadway, Redwood City, Calif. 94062.

Martin P. Conroy, M.D., 108 East Matilija St., Ojai, Calif. 93023.

Norman N. Hoffman, M.D., 9400 Brighton Way, Beverly Hills, Calif. 90210.

Canada:

James K. McGregor, M.D., Medical Arts Building, 174 John St., East Wingham, Ont.

As mentioned earlier, it is best to enclose a *self-addressed, stamped* envelope (or postcard) when communicating by mail with a physician. This will serve the physician's convenience and hasten the reply.

Chapter 16

The Examination

There is a great deal of patient apprehension concerning an examination of the rectal area, which often prevents many persons from seeking proper medical care. This examination can and should be a tolerable affair.

REASONS FOR APPREHENSION

These may vary widely from one patient to another, but the main reasons seem to be an inhibition or an embarrassment about being examined in this area *and* a fear that the hemorrhoids are caused by a more serious disorder.

Inhibition

Some degree of embarrassment is perfectly normal, as most of us are accustomed to a fair amount of privacy when it involves the functioning of the lower bowels. In addition, this particular view of the body is seldom one to be admired. In the words of Dr. E. Aubrey Cox, author of an amusing book (*Bottoms Up*) concerning his experiences as a proctologist:

> Despite its versatility, sensitivity, and delicate structure, and though it has many characteristics, both physical and functional, the anus is devoid of personality.

> Cover the patient with a sheet, which has a hole in it for examination purposes, and I couldn't tell Josephine from Napoleon.[1]

However reassuring it may be, most "rear ends" do look very much the same to the proctologist. Given the 50-percent-plus incidence of hemorrhoids among adults, the presence of a few hemorrhoids is not unusual either.

Another reason for patient hesitation may be the stories told by others who have had either untimely rectal examinations or surgical hemorrhoidectomies. All too frequently, the first opportunity which a proctologist has to examine the hemorrhoid sufferer is when the patient is the victim of a painful, inflamed blood clot. Although medical textbooks advise against a large-instrument examination at the time of this affliction,[2] a few proctologists still perform such an examination. The resulting additional misery which the patient then suffers may be remembered a long time.

Most patients who have experienced surgical removal of hemorrhoids do not have pleasant memories either. This particular subject has been discussed sufficiently in the introductory chapter.

Fear of More Serious Disorder

The fear that a more serious disorder may be the cause of hemorrhoids is often cited as a reason for patient procrastination. Not only are such fears usually unbased, but in the rare instances when a serious problem is present it is certainly self-defeating to avoid medical care.

Chapter 6 provides information concerning methods other than a physical examination for initially detecting a number of serious disorders. One which involves no discomfort or inconvenience is *the stool test*, which requires the patient to take sample smears of feces on three consecutive days. The samples are then brought to the physician's office where a thirty-second test can determine the presence of "hidden blood" within the feces. A positive result may indicate a number of disorders, including ulcers, a malignancy, diverticulosis, a swollen vein of the esophagus, or a number of other blood diseases.

The stool test should be a part of everyone's annual physical. When necessary, the patient should specifically request this test by the family physician. It can be very difficult to initially detect many of the above disorders, even with the use of instruments.

By seeking immediate medical attention for irregularities of the lower bowels (in addition to an annual stool test), we can provide the medical profession a better opportunity to diagnose and treat any disorder in its early stages. It is foolish to do otherwise.

PREPARATION

Before an examination it is proper to cleanse not only the exterior area but also inside the rectum. This is best accomplished with either a suppository enema or a liquid enema, both of which are described in Chapter 13.

A low-residue (fiber) diet is usually recommended the evening before, as this type of meal is less likely to have made much progress into the lower colon by the time of the examination.

The morning of the examination, the patient may be requested to consume only liquids.

POSITIONS

There are two positions commonly used in proctologic practice.

The one which seems to be more frequently utilized is with the patient facedown in what is termed a *knee-chest* position. In those offices equipped with a proctologic table, the patient kneels on a step which is a part of the table, with the chest and abdomen lying on a comfortably padded surface.

The table is then electrically elevated and tilted; and if the table is a true proctologic table, the portion of the table on which the abdomen is resting permits the abdomen to expand without being compressed.

When the knee-chest position is utilized in an office without a proctologic table, the patient customarily kneels on a flat table with the chest down and the buttocks up in the air. With no other support, this can become tiresome and uncomfortable.

Many, but not all, of the proctologists who perform cryotherapy seem to prefer another position called the *left lateral position*. Dr. J. P. Partridge, a well-known British surgeon, suggests this position for the examination of hemorrhoid patients.[3]

In assuming the left lateral position, the patient simply lies on a flat examining table sideways with the left shoulder and hip in contact with the table surface. Patients often find this to be more relaxing than the knee-chest position. Having been examined by both methods, I definitely prefer the left lateral position.

In this more relaxed position it may be easier for the patient to cooperate with the physician during examination. The nerves inside the rectum and lower colon are rather insensitive to ordinary touch, as the mucous-membrane lining has few nerves. This lining is sensitive to stretching though, which makes it important for the patient to relax during the examination. When the patient is not relaxed, the resultant stretching may cause the colon to tighten. This, of course, hampers the examination.

Whichever position is utilized by the cryosurgeon, the patient should remember that this is a very short examination, seldom requiring more than a minute or two.

THE EXAMINATION

The majority of physicians are quite willing to talk their patients through this examination. Sometimes, simply telling the patient what the doctor is doing reduces the patient's tension. Other physicians often carry on a general conversation with their patients. Since the examination involves a sense of discomfort, not pain, it is only necessary to get the patient's mind occupied with other matters in order to reduce this discomfort.

Digital

Initially the physician may make a digital examination, using the index finger to sense the state of the anal canal and the first few inches of the rectal area.

Of course, the physician's glove is adequately lubricated first. This examination is usually conducted with minimal discomfort, even being tolerable in some cases when the patient has a blood clot.

Anoscopy

There are two instruments commonly used to inspect the rectum and lower colon. The first is called an anoscope. It is only three and a half inches long and is used to inspect the lining of the rectum. Upon being warmed to body temperature and properly lubricated, the anoscope is easily introduced and provides a lighted view of the rectal area. This examination is also well tolerated by most patients, since it causes little discomfort.

Sigmoidoscopy

The sigmoidoscope is longer (approximately ten inches) and provides the physician with the most important view of the entire examination.

It is in the lower colon where most colonic malignancies begin, and this instrument can detect their presence. It has a lighted, built-in lens just like the anoscope. The instrument is only one-half the potential dilation of the anal canal and should not cause pain normally.

When the patient cannot relax sufficiently to permit the colon to be viewed, the physician may often pump a bit of air into the lower colon in order to complete the examination. This is preferable to the use of undue pressure, but it does result in some slight discomfort later until the "extra gas" has been passed.

There are several new tests and instruments being developed to make proctologic examinations more tolerable and therefore acceptable to the patient. One of the more promising techniques is the use of fiber optics.[4] This involves the use of a flexible, tube-like viewing instrument which contains two bundles of optical fibers (one bundle to shed a powerful light and the other to carry the magnified image back to the physician). Such an instrument is already available for proctologic examinations. Its advantages are greater flexibility and a longer viewing range.

Dr. David R. Sanderson, associate director of the Lung Project at the Mayo Clinic, has provided the names of two manufacturers of these instruments:

> American Cystoscope Makers, Inc., Attention: Robert Quint, 8 Pelham Parkway, Pelham Park, N.Y. 10803; and
>
> Olympus Corporation of America, Attention: Michael Obstfeld, 2 Nevada Drive, New Hyde Park, N.Y. 11040.

Chapter 17

Cryosurgery

This chapter provides information concerning cryosurgery which a patient might normally be interested in. The Addendum by Dr. Savin (immediately following the chapter) furnishes a detailed medical account of the cryosurgical procedure.

The basis of cryosurgery is cellular destruction by rapid freezing, followed by natural thawing. In comparison with excisional surgery, there is little discomfort or pain. In most cases the patient can expect to return to a normal work routine within a few days. Individuals with less severe hemorrhoids or a higher tolerance for discomfort often return to work the day following the procedure.[1,2,3,4,5]

THE CRYOPROBE

This is the instrument which delivers the freezing temperature to the surface of the hemorrhoidal tissue. There are a variety of instruments in use, most of which utilize either nitrous oxide or liquid nitrogen as the freezing agent. The cryoprobe is a simple instrument, usually a device light enough to be easily held in the physician's hand. The freezing agent circulates through a system of tubes, cooling the tip of the cryoprobe sufficiently to freeze the hemorrhoid. When applied to the hemorrhoid it is placed softly, yet firmly, against the protruding tissue.

VARIOUS CRYOSURGICAL TECHNIQUES

The techniques utilized by cryosurgeons vary; and, consequently, the postoperative course can also be expected to vary somewhat. This chapter will provide information concerning these various methods along with the corresponding postoperative results.

Within or Outside the Anal Canal

Hemorrhoidal tissue may be frozen while it is still within the anal canal *or* in its prolapsed position.[6] Tissue frozen within the anal canal tends to swell less than tissue which is frozen while in the prolapsed position.[7] Therefore, a number of physicians prefer to treat hemorrhoids within the anal canal, as this technique permits the treatment of all hemorrhoids in *one session*. The resultant swelling and anal discomfort is usually quite tolerable.

When hemorrhoids are frozen in their prolapsed position, the increased swelling which follows may cause excessive discomfort. An easy remedy to this problem is simply to schedule treatment over more than one session.[8,9] This reduces the amount of swelling within the anal canal at any one time.

The swelling in either method will result in a certain degree of anal irritation for a few days after treatment.[10] The patient may have a continuing sense of urgency for a bowel movement due to the swelling. In this instance the patient *should not tarry* on the toilet when a bowel movement is not quickly forthcoming. In such circumstances it may be more comforting simply to have a leisurely bath with some enjoyable reading material. Additional relief measures are discussed later in this chapter.

Direct Freezing or Ligation First?

When cryotherapy was initially developed for treating hemorrhoids, there was some difficulty in adequately freezing large prolapsing hemorrhoids.[11]

A number of physicians found that they could effectively freeze these larger hemorrhoids if they ligated the tissue first.[12,13,14] Ligation involves the placement of an elastic band around the base of the hemorrhoid, effectively cutting off the circulation of blood within the ligated tissue.[15,16,17,18] This makes the hemorrhoidal tissue more vulnerable to the freezing temperatures of the cryoprobe. Most cyrosurgeons utilizing this technique freeze only that tissue which lies beneath the mucosal lining of the anal canal.[19]

More recently, other physicians have developed techniques which enable them to effectively *direct-freeze* hemorrhoids without recourse to ligation first.[20,21,22,23,24] The Addendum which follows this chapter describes one physician's technique in detail.

Time Span of Freezes

The length of time in which the cryoprobe is applied to hemorrhoidal tissue has been found to be very important in effectively destroying hemorrhoidal tissue *and* avoiding postoperative complications. This is the case whether the hemorrhoid is directly frozen or ligated first.

Some physicians rely entirely upon the visual appearance of the iceball formation to determine when the tissue has received adequate freezing. After waiting for the iceball to thaw out before repeating the procedure, they again simply watch the size of the iceball to determine the adequacy of the freeze.

There are other physicians, particularly Dr. Savin, who firmly believe that the timing of the freezes is essential to obtain predictable results. Dr. Savin believes that each application of the cryoprobe should be of one-minute duration with the instrument he uses.[25] A number of other physicians also have found that one-minute applications of the cryoprobe to most hemorrhoidal tissues yield the best results.[26,27,28,29,30]

In addition, Dr. Savin strongly advocates that the cryoprobe should be placed along and in direct contact with all the hemorrhoidal tissue to be destroyed.[31] A "Cryodosage Guide" developed for use with his technique appears as Table 3 in the Addendum.

This method of repeated one-minute freezes permits the demarcation between the frozen tissue and the unaffected tissue to be more sharply defined. The eventual result is a smoother separation of the hemorrhoidal tissue from the lining of the anal cushion. This procedure may require a bit more time on the part of the physician, but Dr. Savin reports that the average freezing time of his procedure is only ten minutes per patient.[32]

LOSS OF HEMORRHOIDAL TISSUE

When the hemorrhoids have been properly frozen, the hemorrhoidal tissue will simply fall away from the lining of the anal canal, approximately one to two weeks later.[33,34,35] This falling away (sloughing) of hemorrhoidal tissue will take place most likely during the course of a bowel movement. The sloughing may go unnoticed by the patient unless there is some bleeding at the time. Any bleeding which is noticed should be little more than the slight bleeding experienced during the passage of hard stools prior to cryotherapy.[36,37,38,39] In four to six weeks the skin will regenerate itself, retaining normal pliability and appearance.[40,41,42] Some depigmentation of the new skin occurs.

When hemorrhoids are frozen while in the prolapsed position, there will be an increase in the amount of drainage which may necessitate the use of an absorbent pad for a few weeks. This is also the case when freezing hemorrhoidal tissue which lies beneath the modified anal skin (outer two-thirds of the anal canal), or perianal skin.[43,44,45,46]

YOUR CRYOTHERAPY

The degree of satisfaction a patient experiences after cryotherapy is somewhat dependent upon the preparation prior to treatment. This preparation should include:

1. a proper diet (see Chapters 7 and 8),
2. correct toilet habits (see Chapters 9 and 10), and
3. a thorough understanding of cryotherapy.

Home Preparation

Most physicians will direct the patient to prepare in the same manner as for an examination. Consume a light meal the evening before, and then mostly liquids the day of treatment. A cleansing enema should be taken shortly before going to the physician's office.

Should the physician give the reader different instructions from those suggested in this chapter, follow the doctor's instructions but do not hesitate to ask questions.

Office Interview

At the physician's office, the first step will usually be an interview concerning the symptoms experienced by the patient, along with a description of the physician's procedure.

Many patients will be relieved to find that most cryosurgeons seem to prefer the left lateral position (described in Chapter 16) for their patients during cryosurgery.[47,48,49,50,51]

After determining the course of the medical treatment, the patient is then directed to a room similar to an ordinary examining room. Usually clothing above the waist need not be removed. A towel or sheet is provided.

Desensitizing Agents

The physician's first step is to tell the patient to relax. When the technique employed dictates the use of a desensitizing ointment or local anesthetic, it will be applied at this time. When the proctologist suggests that the use of a desensitizing agent is optional, the patient may state his or her preferences, and should discuss this preference with the physician.

My own cryosurgery did not require an anesthetic. There was some discomfort, which was dissipated by the nurse instructing me to breathe deeply during the applications. During a second session, I was distracted by a conversation with the cryosurgeon. It should be noted that I generally prefer no anesthetic in a dental office either. Again, the use of an anesthetic is first a decision of the physician, and secondly the patient's decision.

Most physicians do apply a desensitizing ointment or a local anesthetic.[52,53,54,55,56]

The Freezing

When the physician and cryoprobe are ready, the patient may be asked to bear down slightly in order to cause the protrusion of the hemorrhoids. A small plastic shield is then used to isolate each prolapsed hemorrhoid for freezing.[57]

Other physicians, who prefer to freeze each hemorrhoid while it remains inside of the anal canal, apply the cryoprobe through a small anoscope (after the anal canal has been desensitized). Since the anal canal is only an inch-and-a-quarter in length, this is a very simple procedure.

When the physician's technique includes ligation, this is swiftly accomplished by the use of a specially designed apparatus.

After the cryoprobe is applied to the hemorrhoidal tissue, a slight stinging sensation is felt—similar to that of holding an ice cube to any other portion of the body. This sensation is only noticed, of course, if no desensitizing agent is present. As mentioned earlier, the degree of discomfort experienced is highly dependent on each individual's tolerance.

The length of time required for the entire procedure will depend on the number and size of the hemorrhoids present, in addition to the cryosurgical technique. Usually, ten to fifteen minutes is all that is required.

At the conclusion of the treatment, the patient may be asked to rest for a short while before leaving the physician's office. It should be noted that frequently the cryosurgery may be performed in hospital facilities, due to either the physician's or patient's preferences. Occasionally, the treatment of hemorrhoids may be combined with another medical procedure.

Postoperative Care

Before leaving the physician's office or hospital, the patient will be given proper instructions to alleviate any discomfort and hasten a return to normal. The physician might prescribe a desensitizing ointment or suppository at this time.[58,59,60,61]

If it is the habit of the patient to consume constipating foods, he or she is well advised to alter this habit during the following six weeks (if not permanently). No alcoholic beverages are advised if the patient should experience severe rectal burning. If patients drink more than three cups of coffee daily, similar discomfort may occur. The amount of citrus juices should be reduced—specifically orange, grapefruit, and tomato juice. Spices such as pepper should also be limited.[62]

It is customary for the patient to use a stool softener during the recovery period. A stool softener is not a laxative, or meant to be, and should be chosen carefully, with the aid of the physician. Some doctors (Canadian and British) recommend the use of unprocessed bran flakes (not commercially advertised breakfast cereals) instead of liquid stool softeners.[63] Unprocessed bran flakes are available in most supermarkets and health-food stores and can be added to blender drinks, cereals, salads, soups, gravies, and many other foods without altering either the taste or appearance of the food.

It would be very intelligent at this time to consume meals rich in fiber content, as described in Chapter 8. The patient can greatly assist recovery without complications by consuming a proper diet.[64] Since the lack of a proper diet may be one of the prime causes of the hemorrhoidal condition in the first place, such a dietary improvement should be considered on a permanent basis.

The physician may also advise short *sitz baths*.[65] These are frequent, warm (not hot) baths in three to four inches of water. They can be taken after each meal for periods of ten minutes.[66]

As mentioned earlier, the patient should expect some anal soreness and also a sense of urgency for a bowel movement due to swelling after cryosurgery. The anal soreness may not become particularly noticeable until the third day or so after treatment. If the soreness is sufficiently severe, an analgesic pill (such as Darvocet-N 100) might be prescribed.[67] The liberal application of Noxzema cream to the anal area may also provide some relief.[68] Applying *two ice cubes in a plastic bag* to the area as frequently as possible within the limits of comfort may also assist.[69]

Most physicians report that fewer than 10 percent of their patients request any form of sedatives during their postoperative period. [70,71,72,73]

Bowel movements are usually accomplished without difficulty, even on the day of cryotherapy.[74,75] The swollen hemorrhoidal tissue may encourage false urges, which can make it difficult to determine when the bowel movement has been completed. When in doubt, get off the toilet!

In a week to ten days the physician may wish to check the progress of the hemorrhoids. At this time the patient is not examined with instruments, as the anal canal is still in the process of regenerating the treated tissue.[76] The necessity of future sessions can be established at this appointment.

The success of cryosurgery depends not only on the efforts of the physician but also on the intelligent preparation and cooperation of the patient. The physician is not in a position to ensure that the patient consumes a proper diet, or does not strain on the toilet. An improvement in these two areas should have occurred well before cryosurgery.

It should be revealed that many patients redevelop hemorrhoids years after various procedures for their removal. Although the new technique of cryotherapy is relatively painless and simple, it is far more intelligent to improve the dietary and toilet habits which have led to hemorrhoidal development and thereby avoid the necessity for repeated medical attention. The information provided in this book should assist in finding permanent relief from this problem.

I hope this book will be a beginning for many people who desire a better understanding of hemorrhoids. Permit me to quote a portion of Dr. Banov's letter:

> A thousand years from now the medical historian might ponder this ironic thought. In its collective wisdom, the United States Government has spent over 50 billion dollars to study the backside of the moon, an area that has caused no one any suffering. But the same government has not spent one cent to study the backsides of its citizens to find out why they suffer from hemorrhoidal disease and what might be done to prevent their painful piles.[77]

Addendum

Hemorrhoidectomy–How I Do It

Results of 444 Cryorectal Surgical Operations
by
Sanford Savin, M.D.

2660 Main Street
Bridgeport, Connecticut
06606
&

Chief of Proctology
Park City Hospital
Bridgeport, Connecticut

(Dr. Savin was a guest speaker and a panelist at a symposium presented at the meeting of the American Society of Colon and Rectal Surgeons in New Orleans, Louisiana —May 1976—at which time this paper was presented.

This report was later published in the April 1977 issue of the medical journal *Diseases of the Colon and Rectum*. It is reprinted by permission of Dr. Savin and J. B. Lippincott Company of Philadelphia, Pennsylvania.)

Cryogenic Rectal Surgery,[1] the application of lethally cold temperatures to unwanted anorectal tissues, when properly employed, permits a one-stage operative procedure for eradication of hemorrhoids, internal and external, and related anorectal disorders.

A cryosurgical method for the eradication of hemorrhoids was first introduced in 1969.[2] In the intervening years, additional publications have offered a variety of methods for employing cryosurgery for the treatment of hemorrhoids.[1-11]

In 1974, this author[10] reported to the American Society of Colon and Rectal Surgeons on the excellent early results obtained in the first 145 operations of this current series in which not only combined hemorrhoids but all associated anorectal pathologic conditions were managed in one stage.

The series now consists of 444 cryorectal operations and longer-term observations.

All cryosurgical operations in this series were performed with the KRYmed FT-300 fixed-tip cryosurgical probe for proctology. The KRYmed FT-300 with the T-0832 crysurgical probe is manufactured by Cryomedics Incorporated, of Bridgeport, Connecticut. The rectangular cryotip is 32 mm long and 8 mm wide and is permanently fitted to an insulated shaft. The cryotip is made of hollowed coin silver to provide maximum thermoconductivity. Optimum results are achieved by applying the dry, flat surface of the cryotip to moistened target tissue to gain maximum surface contact and then precisely timing the freeze. The KRYmed FT-300 probe has a pistol-grip and trigger. The probe is attached by tubing to a cylinder of nitrous oxide. Squeezing the trigger permits nitrous oxide to flow through the hollowed cryotip, actuating a freeze cycle. Release of the trigger effects instant cryotip defrost. The gas exits from a remote exhaust.

CONDITIONS TREATED (1973-1975)

The surgical objective has been the eradication of all grades and types of hemorrhoids and concomitant pathologic conditions in one operative session. The primary indication for cryorectal surgery in all 444 cases was bleeding, painful or prolapsing hemorrhoids, either internal, or internal and external. Forty-four per cent of the patients examined were found to have concomitant anorectal pathologic conditions (Table 1).

Table 1. Conditions Treated

HEMORRHOIDS, INTERNAL AND EXTERNAL		444
Concomitant conditions		
Fissure-in-ano	89	
Fistula-in-ano	30	
Hypertrophied anal papillae	44	
Fibrous polyps	19	
Condylomata acuminata	8	
Mucosal prolapse	3	
Miscellaneous	2	
	195	
		(44 percent)

In addition to hemorrhoids, cryosurgery was used for fissures, hypertrophied anal papillae, condylomas, rectal mucosal prolapse, and miscellaneous benign lesions. Fistulectomies, fibrous polypectomies, and some fissurectomies were by excision (Table 2).

Table 2. Concomitant Operations Performed during Cryohemorrhoidectomy

CRYODESTRUCTIONS		EXCISIONS	
Anal fissure	80	Anal fissure	9
Anal fistula	1	Anal fistula	29
Hypertrophied anal papillae	44	Fibrous polyps	19
Condylomata acuminata	8		57
Mucosal prolapse	3		
Miscellaneous	2		
	138		

Initially, cryorectal surgery was offered with caution as an optional method of hemorrhoidectomy but, with increasing confidence in technique and results, it was offered as the procedure of choice.

There were 276 male and 168 female patients, ranging in

age from 17 to 78 years. All were screened with the customary examinations: endoscopy, laboratory work and x-rays when indicated. Patients were not excluded for medical reasons, and 47 of them had serious concurrent problems. Such poor operative candidates as cardiac and diabetic patients and those who had terminal renal disease were operated upon with minimal risk by this method.

OPERATIVE MANAGEMENT

Patients are advised that their anorectal disease will receive a definitive freezing treatment in a one-stage operation so that they will suffer less pain and dysfunction than might be anticipated after excisional hemorrhoidectomy.

Although the operation may be performed either in the hospital or in the office, the actual decision for or against hospitalization depends upon the medical condition of the patient and his family needs and desires. By mutual agreement, 331 (66 per cent) were hospitalized, and 113 (34 per cent) had the procedure in the office.

Preoperative cleansing enemas are ordered. The patient is placed in the left lateral position on the operating table with the buttocks strapped apart. The perianal area is scrubbed and then painted with povidone-iodine solution. In the office, diazepam, 7.5 mg, is administered intramuscularly. In the hospital, the anesthetist selects a suitable tranquilizer. Local anesthesia consisting of 10 ml of 2 per cent lidocaine is administered subcutaneously throughout the perianal area, and then a deep injection of 10 ml bupivacaine 0.25 per cent, is made by placing 2.5 ml in each quadrant outside the rectal wall with a finger in the rectum as a guide. Prior to the freezing of external hemorrhoids a third anesthetic (10 ml of 0.25% bupivacaine) is deposited subcutaneously around the perianal area. This is to eliminate or reduce the possibility of post-thaw burning, which can be quite severe. On rare occasions, general anesthesia is administered upon request.

A right-angle open-sided retractor is used for exposure of

the internal hemorrhoidal mass and, when necessary, the external hemorrhoid is grasped with an Allis clamp to improve exposure and produce tension. The flat side of the rectangular cryotip is placed longitudinally in firm contact with the long axis of a segment of the internal hemorrhoid. Squeezing the trigger actuates the freezing process; in seconds the tissue adheres to the probe. The cryotip is now elevated and the predetermined dosage administered (Table 3). As each freeze is administered, the time and anatomic location of treatment are recorded.

Table 3 Cryodosage Guide *
(KRY med FT-300 with T-0832)

	FREEZE TIME PER APPLICATION *(Minutes)*
Hemorrhoid, internal	1–1½
Hemorrhoid, external	1½–3
Anal fissure	½–1
Hypertrophied anal papillae	½–1½
Condylomata acuminata	⅙–1½
Mucosal prolapse	2

* Determined empirically. Operating pressure = 645 to 800 psi. Refrigerant = nitrous oxide.

Releasing the probe trigger actuates defrosting and the cryotip is instantly free of the tissue. Only tissue directly beneath the cryotip should be the target. For this reason, *separate applications* are made to segmental portions of the internal hemorrhoids until every area has been directly frozen. In this fashion, each internal hemorrhoidal mass will have received an average dosage of 2 to 3 minutes freezing.

Particular care is taken with external hemorrhoids. Direct contact freezing of external hemorrhoids and redundant perianal skin is done without attempting to preserve perianal skin islands. The cryodosage per application ranges from 1½ to 3 minutes, depending upon the size and mass of the external hemorrhoids. Similarly, any area involved by a concomitant pathologic condition is frozen separately, with varying dosages. When excisional surgery is performed, it precedes the freezing. A repeat freeze-thaw-freeze-thaw cycle is useful instead of prolonged freezing for unusually large thickened masses.

Overzealous or inadequate freezing increases the risk of complications and poor results. Knowledge of the full extent of the pathologic condition is mandatory, as the latent process of cryodestruction, once initiated, is irreversible.

Perianal skin becomes more edematous than mucosa when subjected to thermal insult. To reduce this effect, the swollen skin is thoroughly massaged to express serum.

Following the cryosurgical procedure, the rectal pouch and perianal skin are again painted with providone-iodine to inhibit bacterial growth, and absorbent dressings are applied.

Office patients are kept at rest for approximately 30 minutes with monitoring of vital signs before being allowed to leave, with escort. Hospital patients go through regular recovery room procedure.

POSTOPERATIVE MANAGEMENT

Management of the patients after operation consists of frequent changes of dressings, prescribing stool-softener laxatives, a regular diet without spices and alcohol, and an analgesic, if needed, for discomfort. Immediate ambulation of the patient, painless bowel movements, and resumption of normal activities are anticipated.

Office visits are recommended one, three and six weeks after cryosurgery, after which time most patients are healed. Early digital or instrumental examination of the rectal outlet is not necessary. Some patients are discharged in less than three weeks, but 48 patients took more than two months for complete healing, and most of those had also been treated for fissure or excision of anal fistulas, which contributed to the delays.

At the first postoperative visit, the patient is interrogated to elicit possible complaints, and advice is given when necessary. The postoperative instructions are reviewed with the patient again, and the operative site is examined. When there is a significant amount of slough, it is trimmed away. At the three-week visit, the patient is again interviewed; the wounds are inspected, alterations may be made in diet, medication, and home care. At six weeks, at which time most patients are fully healed, a digital examination is performed, followed by anoscopy, to evaluate the results.

POSTOPERATIVE COURSE

The process of cryodestruction and repair goes through several stages. Immediately after cryosurgery the tissues appear bluish, engorged, and somewhat edematous, representing vascular stasis and ischemia. Edema is most marked when large external hemorrhoids have been treated; otherwise, it is minimal or absent. The edema dissipates within 48 hours as serosanguineous drainage. The insulted tissues undergo infarction, the prior swellings feel indurated, and the drainage becomes whitish. During these stages, patients may complain of rectal pressure and tenesmus.

The infarcted area starts to undergo necrotic change and bacterial colonization, if not inhibited, may result in odor and purulent discharge. These changes begin approximately three to four days after operation, during which time patients may experience rectal burning or soreness. These symptoms are usually relieved with simple measures.

The necrotic tissue is sharply demarcated and sloughs away gradually within one to two weeks, leaving a thin layer of granulation tissue covering the wounds. Epithelialization completes the process, without scar tissue contraction, in about six weeks.

None of the postoperative complications listed in Table 4 is statistically significant; however, an attempt is made to evaluate the cause and possible prevention of each.

Ten patients requested an injection for pain in the hospital or took a prescribed narcotic orally at home. It was difficult to determine whether they had true pain, rectal pressure, apprehension, or combinations of factors.

Eight patients of the 444 complained of intense pain and suffering for two to three weeks. Each case was carefully analyzed. Four of these patients had had cryodestruction of internal hemorrhoids and electrodesiccation of external hemorrhoids as a clinical trial. This experience led to the discarding of electrodesiccation. Three of the patients were judged to have had improper freezing technique. The eighth patient had slight stenosis of the anal canal causing severe constipation and distress. His pain was promptly relieved by dilatations in the office when the condition was discovered.

Urinary retention occurred in seven patients, but was unique because it did not develop until the second to seventh postoperative days. In one patient in the group, transurethral resection was necessary.

Table 4. Postoperative Complications of Cryorectal Surgery, 444 Patients (1973-1975)

Condition		Number
Pain		
Less than 48 hours	10	
Prolonged	8	
		18
Urinary retention		7
Hemorrhage		
Secondary—		
Stopped spontaneously	12	
Required treatment	6	
		18
Fecal impaction		5

Twelve patients mentioned a gush of blood or bleeding of bright red blood per rectum occurring between the ninth and twenty-first postoperative days, coinciding with the final slough of hemorrhoids. This bleeding stopped spontaneously or responded to treatment with bed rest and application of ice packs to the area.

Secondary hemorrhage necessitating surgical intervention occurred in six patients between the ninth and nineteeth days after operation. Only one of these six patients needed a blood transfusion.

Five of the hemorrhages occurred in the first year of the series; only one has occurred subsequently.

Fecal impaction was reported five times, and was probably the result of fear to strain down sufficiently to evacuate the rectal pouch. These five patients required manual break-up of the impaction and the use of oil retention enemas. Subsequently they had no difficulty with their bowel movements.

Fever, inguinal node swelling, itching, fecal soiling, anorexia, loss of anal canal sensation and perianal and buttocks rash were also reported, but did not require special treatment and were statistically insignificant.

Among the residual postoperative findings, perianal depigmentation occurred in nine patients, none of whom was Caucasian. Fistula from bridging was found in three patients.

Perianal skin tags were recorded as occurring in 106 patients (24 per cent). It was found that in the first year of this series 31 per cent of the patients had persistent skin tags, and in the second year, with a change in technique, a 21 per cent incidence was reported. This is a substantial 33 per cent reduction in overall incidence (Table 5). Current operative technique has successfully avoided the problem.

Table 5. Effect of Change in Technique on Skin Tag Formation

Year	Number of Patients	Skin Tags Number	Skin Tags Per Cent
1973–74	139	43	31
1974–75	295	63	21

When the series of cryosurgical hemorrhoidectomies was begun, simultaneous freezing of an internal-external hemorrhoid with a single prolonged freeze of at least 3 minutes' duration was employed. This technique resulted in the highest percentage of skin tag formation and secondary hemorrhage.

The current freezing technique used is direct-contact freezing of each internal hemorrhoidal complex in segments, with preservation of adjacent mucosa, followed by direct-contact freezing of all external hemorrhoidal tissue and redundant perianal skin without attempting to preserve skin islands. The freeze times used in this technique adhere to the Cryodosage Guide (Table 3). This has practically eliminated the formation of postoperative skin tags and has not resulted in stricture or other problems.

POSTOPERATIVE RESULTS (SHORT-TERM)

Excellent results were obtained in eliminating all hemorrhoids and symptoms in 431 of 434 patients, or a 99 per cent cure rate. Ten patients were lost to follow-up and three patients had some residual hemorrhoidal tissue.

Cryodestruction was successful in removing 97 per cent of the concomitant pathologic conditions treated (Table 6).

Table 6. Short-term Operative Results of 444 Cryorectal Operations (1973-1975)

	Patients	Successes	Failures
Cryohemorrhoidectomies			
Internal and external	444 *	431	(Partial) 3
Concomitant cryodestructions			
Anal fissure	80	78	2
Anal fistula	1	1	0
Hypertrophic anal papillae	44	42	2
Condylomata acuminata	8	8	0
Mucosal prolapse	3	3	0
Miscellaneous	2	2	0

* Ten patients lost to follow-up.

POSTOPERATIVE RESULTS (LONG-TERM)

Two hundred sixty-seven patients were examined six months after operation (Table 7). All patients were asymptomatic, and 261 had no objective evidence of disease, representing a 98 per cent success rate.

Table 7. Long-term Results (Recurrences) in Cryohemorrhoidectomies (1973-1975)

Postoperative Period	Patients Examined	Hemorrhoids Internal	Hemorrhoids External	Combined Hemorrhoids
6–9 months	267	5	1	0
1–2 years	155	3	1	0
2–3 years	44	1	0	1

Five were found to have single asymptomatic internal hemorrhoids. One had an external hemorrhoid. Three patients, all from the group previously treated for fissures, had fissures. Two patients were found to have recurrent condylomas. The same two patients still had hypertrophic anal papillae (Table 8).

Table 8. Long-term Results (Recurrences) in Cryorectal Surgical Procedures for Treatment of Concomitant Pathologic Conditions (1973-1975)

Condition	Number	6–9 Months	1–2 Years	2–3 Years
Anal fissure	80	3	1	0
Anal fistula	1	0	0	0
Hypertrophic anal papillae	44	2	5	1
Condylomata acuminata	8	2	0	1
Mucosal prolapse	3	0	0	0
Miscellaneous	2	0	0	0

One hundred fifty-five patients were evaluated one to two years after operation. One hundred fifty-one patients were graded as having excellent results. Three patients had asymptomatic internal varices, small in size; one had an external hemorrhoid. Three patients were found to have hypertrophic anal papillae not present before. Two patients still had the persistent hypertrophic anal papillae.

The longest follow-up period in the series was two to three years. Forty-four patients in this category were examined, and 42 were considered to have excellent results. One patient had an internal hemorrhoid not present at the six-month examination and, therefore, regarded as a recurrence. One patient was found to have internal and external hemorrhoids requiring additional treatment that had not been present at the end of six months and one year. One patient treated for condylomas was free of disease at the end of six months and one year, but condylomas were found at the end of two years. One patient had hypertrophic anal papillae not present before.

In all categories, there was a 98 per cent cure rate on long-term follow-up.

DISCUSSION

Postoperative pain associated with excisional hemorrhoidectomy is not universal, but occurs with such frequency as to discourage many sufferers from seeking diagnosis and treatment for their rectal ailments.

These factors have led to acceptance of sclerotherapy and more recently, internal ligation of hemorrhoids, which are, at best, incomplete treatments with their own complications. Cryorectal surgery offers the opportunity to perform a definitive complete operation for both internal and external hemorrhoids and all *concomitant* pathologic conditions. The results over a three-year period, both short- and long-term, have been excellent. While it is true that radical cryohemorrhoidectomy produces more patient inconveniences than sclerotherapy or internal ligations, on the other hand, it eradicates all the diseased tissue in one procedure, and has much less painful consequences than excisional surgery.

Some surgeons [3,4,7-10] reporting successful results with cryohemorrhoidectomy limit the types of hemorrhoids treated and supplement direct-contact freezing with internal ligations. The cryosurgical technique employed for the 444 patients in this series seems to overcome the problems encountered by others.

CONCLUSIONS

Based on a three-year personal experience with a large number of patients, cryorectal surgery is a reliable and valuable alternative to excision for the removal of all types of hemorrhoids and most other concomitant pathologic conditions found in 44 per cent of these patients. Excellent results should be anticipated, and complications are minimal. No contraindication has yet been detected.

Notes

CHAPTER 1

1. J. C. Goligher, M.D., *Surgery of the Anus, Rectum, and Colon,* Second Edition (Springfield, Illinois: Charles C. Thomas, 1967), p. 111.

2. Marvin L. Corman, M.D., Malcolm C. Veidenheimer, M.D., and John A. Coller, M.D., "Alternatives of Surgical Hemorrhoidectomy," *Geriatrics,* October 1974, p. 99.

3. Denis P. Burkitt, M.D., "Varicose Veins, Deep Vein Thrombosis, and Haemorrhoids: Epidemiology, and Suggested Aetiology," *British Medical Journal,* Volume 2, June 3, 1972, p. 556.

4. Article, "Phlebology: Palliatives But No Cures," *Time,* January 13, 1967.

5. Louis A. Buie, Sr., M.D., *Practical Proctology,* Second Edition (Springfield, Illinois: Charles C. Thomas, 1960), p. 219.

6. Robert T. Turell, M.D., *Diseases of the Colon and Anorectum,* Volume II (Philadelphia: W. B. Saunders, 1969), p. 843.

7. See Note 5.

8. Article, "By Non-Surgical Treatment, Hemorrhoid Operations Reduced 75%," *Santa Ana Register,* October 14, 1976.

9. James A. Ferguson, M.D., "Diverse Methods of Managing Hemorrhoids: Surgical Treatment," *Diseases of the Colon and Anorectum,* May–June 1973, p. 173.

10. Lyon Hyams, M.D., and John Philpot, Ph.D., "An Epidemiological Investigation of Hemorrhoids," *American Journal of Proctology,* June 1970, p. 177.

11. Martin I. Lewis, M.D., "A Cryosurgical Hemorrhoidectomy: A Follow-up Report," *Diseases of the Colon and Rectum,* March–April 1972, p. 128.

12. Lawrence Goldbacher, M.D., *Hemorrhoids, The Injection Treatment and Pruritus Ani* (Philadelphia: Davis Company, 1930), p. 35.

13. Thaddeus S. Grosicki, Ph.D., and K. Richard Knoll, Ph.D., *Handbook of Non-Prescription Drugs,* 1973 Edition (Washington, D.C.: American Pharmaceutical Association), p. 133.

14. See Note 12.

15. Denis P. Burkitt, M.D., and H. C. Trowell, M.D., *Refined Carbohydrate Foods and Diseases: Some Implications of Dietary Fibre* (London: Academic Press, 1975), p. 44.

16. See Note 12.

17. Barry Kramer, "Medical Advances: Some New Cures Help Hemorrhoid Sufferers, Whose Number is Legion," *The Wall Street Journal,* August 10, 1973.

18. Emil Ludwig, *Napoleon* (New York: Boni and Liveright, 1926), p. 394.

19. See Note 12.

20. William A. Nolan, M.D., "To Operate or Not: Patient's Choice," *McCall's,* February 1974, p. 80.

21. R. Ross, M.D., "What a Doctor Says You Should Know About Constipation and Hemorrhoids," *Vogue,* May 1976, p. 18.

22. See Note 11.

23. See Note 11, p. 133.

24. Salvatore J. Detrano, M.D., "Cryosurgical Hemorrhoidectomy," *Contemporary Surgery,* September 1973.

25. Sanford Savin, M.D., "The Role of Cryosurgery in Management of Anorectal Disease: Preliminary Report on Results," *Diseases of the Colon and Rectum,* May–June 1975, p. 296.

26. Changyul Oh, M.D., and David A. Dreiling, M.D., "Cryo-Hemorrhoidectomy," *Mt. Sinai Journal of Medicine,* October 1974, p. 658.

27. See Note 13, p. 136.

28. R.E.B. Tagart, M.D., "Haemorrhoids and Palpable Ano-Rectal Lesions," *The Practitioner,* February 1974, p. 222.

29. Joseph Franklin Montague, M.D., *The Modern Treatment of Hemorrhoids* (Philadelphia: J. B. Lippincott, 1926), p. 120.

30. See Note 15, pp. 339–343.

31. William H. Olmsted, M.D., Ray D. Williams, M.D., and Theodore Bauerlein, M.D., "Constipation: The Laxative Value of Bulky Foods," *Medical Clinics of North America,* September 1936, pp. 449–459.

32. See Note 29, pp. 118–120.

33. Denis P. Burkitt, M.D., A. R. P. Walker, M.D., and Neil S. Painter, M.D, "Dietary Fiber and Diseases," *Journal of the American Medical Association*, August 19, 1974, p. 1068.

34. Neil S. Painter, M.D., Anthony Z. Almedida, M.D., and

Kenneth W. Colebourne, M.D., "Unprocessed Bran in Treatment of Diverticular Disease," *British Medical Journal,* April 15, 1972, p. 137.

35. Denis P. Burkitt, M.D., and C. W. Graham-Stewart, M.D., "Haemorrhoids: Postulated Pathogenesis and Proposed Prevention," *Postgraduate Medical Journal,* September 1975, p. 631.

36. Leon Banov, Jr., M.D., "Backsides," *Archives of Surgery,* December, 1974, p. 44.

37. Harold J. Taub, *Keeping Healthy in a Polluted World* (New York: Harper and Row, 1974), pp. 136–137.

38. Hamish Thomson, "Piles, Their Nature and Management," *The Lancet,* September 13, 1975, p. 494.

39. See Note 38.

40. Robert T. Turell, M.D., *Diseases of the Colon and Anorectum,* Volume II (Philadelphia: W. B. Saunders, 1969), p. 906.

41. See Note 38.

42. See Note 28.

43. See Note 38.

44. See Note 1, p. 118.

45. William W. Slack, M.D., "The Problem of Haemorrhoids," *The Practitioner,* November 1969, p. 606.

46. D. P. Burkitt, M.D., "Two Blind Spots In Medical Knowledge," *Nursing Times,* January 8, 1976, pp. 24–27.

47. Denis P. Burkitt, M.D., "Hemorrhoids, Varicose Veins, and Deep Vein Thrombosis: Epidemiologic Features and Suggested Causative Factors," *Canadian Journal of Surgery,* September 1975, p. 483.

48. See Note 29, pp. 118, 119.

49. See Note 24.

50. See Note 28, p. 221.

51. See Note 17.

52. See Note 2, p. 100.

53. See Note 11.

54. J. P. Partridge, M.D., "Treatment of Haemorrhoids," *Nursing Times,* June 12, 1975, p. 929.

55. See Note 11.

56. Changyul Oh, M.D., "Treatment of Hemorrhoids and Applications of Cryotechnique," *Mt. Sinai Journal of Medicine,* March 1974, p. 201.

57. John J. O'Connor, M.D., "A Study of Cryosurgical Tech-

niques," *Diseases of the Colon and Rectum,* May–June 1975, p. 299.

58. See Note 2.

59. See Note 17.

60. A. Walsh Low, "Pain in Hemorrhoid Repair," *Nursing Times,* June 12, 1975, p. 930.

61. See Note 8.

62. See Note 8.

63. See Note 8.

64. Personal Communication, Sanford Savin, M.D., June 20, 1977, p. 3.

65. Eugene P. Salvati, M.D., "Symposium: Treatment of Hemorrhoids and Fissures," *Contemporary Surgery,* November 1973, p. 104.

66. Arthur A. Rand, M.D., "Symposium: Treatment of Hemorrhoids and Fissures," *Contemporary Surgery,* November 1973, p. 106.

67. See Note 54.

68. Martin I. Lewis, M.D., "Cryosurgical Hemorrhoidectomy: Preliminary Report," *Diseases of the Colon and Rectum,* September–October 1969, p. 371.

69. See Note 11, p. 134.

70. See Note 56, p. 199.

71. See Note 65, pp. 374, 377, 378.

72. Personal Communication, Sanford Savin, M.D., August 2, 1977.

73. See Note 26, p. 663.

CHAPTER 2

1. William H. Olmsted, M.D., Ray D. Williams, M.D., and Theodore Bauerlein, M.D., "Constipation: The Laxative Value of Bulky Foods," *Medical Clinics of North America,* September 1936, p. 454.

2. Denis P. Burkitt, M.D., and C. W. Graham-Stewart, M.D., "Hemorrhoids—Postulated Pathogenesis and Proposed Prevention," *Postgraduate Medical Journal,* September 1975, p. 633.

3. Robert T. Turell, M.D., *Diseases of the Colon and Anorec-*

tum, Second Edition, Volume II (Philadelphia: W. B. Saunders Company, 1969), p. 916.

4. W. H. F. Thomson, M.D., *British Journal of Surgery,* Volume 62, 1975, p. 542.

5. A. F. Pineda, M.D., "The Importance of Arterial Irrigation in Hemorrhoid Pathology," *American Journal of Proctology,* June 1972, p. 209.

6. Hamish Thomson, M.D., "Piles: Their Nature and Management," *The Lancet,* September 13, 1975, p. 494.

7. See Note 5.

8. See Note 6.

9. D. P. Burkitt, M.D., "Two Blind Spots in Medical Knowledge," *Nursing Times,* January 18, 1976, p. 26.

10. Roy C. Darlington, Ph.D., "Laxatives," *Handbook of Non-Prescription Drugs,* 1973 Edition (Washington, D.C.: American Pharmaceutical Association), p. 55.

11. See Note 10.

12. See Note 2.

CHAPTER 3

1. Peter H. Lord, M.D., "Hemorrhoids—The Dilation Procedure," *Nursing Times,* June 19, 1975, p. 961.

2. D. P. Burkitt, M.D., "Dietary Fibre and Pressure Diseases," *Journal of the Royal College of Physicians,* Volume 9, No. 2, January 1975, p. 143.

3. R. E. B. Tagart, M.D., "Hemorrhoids and Palpable Anorectal Lesions," *The Practitioner,* Volume 212, February 1974, p. 222.

4. W. H. F. Thomson, M.D., *British Journal of Surgery,* 1975, Volume 62, p. 542.

5. O. C. Goss, M.D., and J. Adams, M.D., *American Journal of Surgery,* 1950, Volume 79, p. 40.

6. D. P. Burkitt, M.D., and C. W. Graham-Stewart, M.D., "Hemorrhoids—Postulated Pathogenesis and Proposed Prevention," *Postgraduate Medical Journal,* Volume 51, September 1975, p. 633.

7. Louis A. Buie, Sr., M.D., *Practical Proctology,* Second Edition (Springfield, Illinois: Charles C. Thomas, 1960), p. 219.

CHAPTER 4

1. J. P. Partridge, M.D., "Treatment of Hemorrhoids," *Nursing Times,* June 12, 1975, p. 928.

2. Mandel Ganchrow, M.D., et al., "Thrombosed Hemorrhoids: A Clinical Pathologic Study," *Diseases of the Colon and Rectum,* September 1971, p. 331.

3. Robert T. Turell, M.D., *Diseases of the Colon and Anorectum, Volume II* (Philadelphia: W. B. Saunders, 1969), p. 895.

4. See Note 2.

5. J. C. Goligher, M.D., *Surgery of the Anus, Rectum, and Colon,* Second Edition (Springfield, Illinois: Charles C. Thomas, 1967), p. 117.

6. R. E. B. Tagart, M.D., "Hemorrhoids and Palpable Anorectal Lesions," *The Practitioner,* February 1974, p. 224.

7. See Note 3, p. 907.

8. See Note 6.

9. See Note 7.

10. See Note 5, p. 118.

11. See Note 7.

12. Sanford Savin, M.D., Personal Communication, June 20, 1977, p. 1.

13. See Note 12, p. 2.

14. See Note 12, p. 2.

15. Thaddeus S. Grosicki, Ph.D., and K. Richard Knoll, Ph.D., "Hemorrhoidal Preparations," *Handbook of Non-Prescription Drugs,* 1973 Edition (Washington, D.C.: American Pharmaceutical Association), p. 153.

16. The Editors of Consumer Reports, *The Medicine Show* (New York: Pantheon Books, 1971), p. 76.

17. See Note 7.

18. Barry Kramer, "Medical Advances: Some New Cures Help Hemorrhoidal Sufferers, Whose Number is Legion," *The Wall Street Journal,* August 10, 1973.

CHAPTER 5

1. Robert Terrell, M.D., and James Ferguson, M.D., "Diverse Methods of Managing Hemorrhoids," *Diseases of the Colon and Rectum,* May–June 1973, p. 192.

2. Robert Terrell, M.D., *American Journal of Surgery,* Volume 123, No. 3.

3. D. P. Burkitt, M.D., "Dietary Fibre and Pressure Diseases," *Journal of Royal College of Physicians,* Volume 9, No. 2, January 1975, p. 138.

4. D. P. Burkitt, M.D., and C. W. Graham-Stewart, M.D., "Hemorrhoids—Postulated Pathogenesis and Proposed Prevention," *Postgraduate Medical Journal,* September 1975, p. 632.

5. See Note 4.

6. Joseph Franklin Montague, M.D., *The Modern Treatment of Hemorrhoids* (Philadelphia: J. B. Lippincott, 1926), p. 120.

7. See Note 4, p. 635.

8. R. E. B. Tagart, M.D., "Haemorrhoids and Palpable Anorectal Lesions," *The Practitioner,* February 1974, p. 229.

9. See Note 6, p. 118.

10. See Note 4, p. 635.

11. Denis P. Burkitt, M.D., "Hemorrhoids . . . And Suggested Causative Factors," *Canadian Journal of Surgery,* September 1975, p. 483.

12. Barry Kramer, "Medical Advances: Some New Cures Help Hemorrhoid Sufferers, Whose Number Is Legion," *The Wall Street Journal,* August 10, 1973.

13. See Note 3, p. 145.

14. Denis P. Burkitt, M.D., "Varicose Veins, Deep Vein Thrombosis, and Haemorrhoids: Epidemiology and Suggested Aetiology," *British Medical Journal,* Volume 2, June 3, 1972, p. 559.

15. Neil S. Painter, M.D., "Diverticular Disease of the Colon . . . ," *Geriatrics,* February 1976, p. 90.

16. See Note 15, p. 91.

17. See Note 14, p. 557.

18. See Note 17.

19. See Note 14, p. 558.

20. O. O. Ajayi, M.D., "Anal Fissures, Fistulas, Abscesses, and Hemorrhoids in a Tropical Population," *Diseases of the Colon and Rectum,* January–February 1974, p. 59.

21. See Note 8, p. 222.

22. Lyon Hyams, M.D., and John Philpot, Ph.D., "An Epidemiological Investigation of Hemorrhoids," *American Journal of Proctology,* June 1970, p. 192.

23. See Note 4, p. 631.

24. See Note 11, p. 485.
25. See Note 8, p. 222.
26. See Note 20, p. 57.
27. See Note 14, p. 556.
28. See Note 14, p. 557.
29. See Note 28.
30. See Note 3.
31. See Note 15, p. 89.
32. See Note 14, p. 485.
33. See Note 15, p. 91.
34. See Note 33.
35. See Note 33.
36. See Note 33.
37. See Note 33.
38. See Note 33.
39. Roy C. Darlington, Ph.D., "Laxatives," *Handbook of Non-Prescription Drugs,* 1973 Edition (Washington, D.C.: American Pharmaceutical Association), p. 55.
40. Louis A. Buie, M.D., *Practical Proctology,* Second Edition (Springfield: Charles C. Thomas, 1960), p. 220.
41. See Note 39.
42. G. C. Prasad, M.D., "Studies of Etiopathogenesis of Hemorrhoids," *American Journal of Proctology,* June 1976, p. 36.
43. J. C. Goligher, M.D., *Surgery of the Anus, Rectum, and Colon,* Second Edition (Springfield, Illinois: Charles C. Thomas, 1967), p. 114.
44. Robert E. Rothenberg, M.D., *Understanding Surgery* (New York: Trident Press, 1965), p. 271.
45. See Note 6, p. 119.
46. Marion C. Pruitt, M.D., *Hemorrhoids* (St. Louis: The C. V. Mosby Company, 1938), p. 62.
47. Thaddeus S. Grosicki, Ph.D., and K. Richard Knoll, Ph.D., *Handbook of Non-Prescription Drugs,* 1973 Edition (Washington, D.C.: American Pharmaceutical Association), p. 134.
48. See Note 6, p. 118.
49. Robert T. Turell, M.D., *Diseases of the Colon and Anorectum,* Volume II (Philadelphia: W. B. Saunders, 1969), p. 903.
50. See Note 40, p. 219.
51. See Note 6.

52. See Note 22.

53. Richard T. Shackleford, M.D., *Diseases of the Colon and Anorectum,* Volume II (Philadelphia: W. B. Saunders, 1959), pp. 849, 857.

54. See Note 4, p. 633.

55. See Note 20, p. 55.

CHAPTER 6

1. Louis A. Buie, Sr., M.D., *Practical Proctology,* Second Edition (Springfield, Illinois: Charles C. Thomas, 1960), p. 226.

2. E. Aubrey Cox, M.D., *Bottoms Up* (Durham, North Carolina: Moore Publishing Company, 1969), p. 19.

3. Richard T. Shackleford, M.D., "Hemorrhoids and Their Surgical Treatment," *Diseases of the Colon and Anorectum,* Volume II (Philadelphia: W. B. Saunders, 1969), p. 906.

4. Staff Reporter, "New Methods for Detecting Colon-Rectal Cancer Used," *The Wall Street Journal,* August 15, 1976.

5. See Note 4.

6. R. E. B. Tagart, M.D., "Haemorrhoids and Palpable Ano-Rectal Lesions," *The Practitioner,* February 1974, p. 223.

CHAPTER 7

1. Neil S. Painter, M.D., *British Medical Journal,* Vol. II, 1972, p. 137.

2. Joan Jennings, "Bran Wards Off The Bane Of Elders," *Prevention,* March 1976, p. 210.

3. Denis P. Burkitt, M.D., "Some Diseases Characteristic of Modern Western Civilization," *Clinical Radiology,* Vol. 24, 1973, pp. 271, 272.

4. See Notes 1, 2, and 3.

5. Carl I. Flath, *The Miracle Nutrient* (New York: Bantam, 1976), p. 48.

6. See Note 5, p. 49.

7. See Note 6.

8. See Note 5, p. 50.

9. I. Taylor, M.D., and H. L. Duthie, M.D., "Bran Tablets and

Diverticular Disease," *British Medical Journal,* April 24, 1976, p. 988.

10. See Note 1.

11. Neil S. Painter, M.D., "Diverticular Disease of the Colon: A Bane of the Elderly," *Geriatrics,* February 1976, p. 91.

12. See Note 5, p. 51.

13. D. P. Burkitt, M.D., "Dietary Fibre and Pressure Diseases," *Journal of the Royal College of Physicians (London),* Vol. 9, No. 2, January 1975, p. 146.

14. See Note 5, p. 56.

15. See Note 5, p. 50.

16. See Note 5, p. 66.

17. Shela W. Bordin and Gerald M. Bordin, M.D., "Bran: Roughage That's Rough on Iron," *New England Journal of Medicine,* January 1, 1976, p. 57.

CHAPTER 8

1. Sumner C. Kraft, M.D., *The Trans/Vision Book of Health* (London: Helen H. Benton, 1974), p. 74.

2. S. Weir Newmayer, M.D., and Edwin C. Broome, Ph.D., *Health in Good-Habit Land* (New York: American Book Company, 1934), pp. 25–28.

3. A. R. P. Walker, M.D., F. W. Fox, M.D., and J. T. Irving, M.D., *Biochemistry Journal,* Vol. 42, 1948, p. 452.

4. Article, *Los Angeles Times,* January 5, 1977, p. 7.

5. Article, *Los Angeles Times,* February 2, 1977, p. 3.

6. See Note 4.

7. See Note 4.

8. Article, *Los Angeles Times,* February 17, 1977, p. 7.

9. See Note 1, pp. 76, 81.

10. D. P. Burkitt, M.D., and H. C. Trowell, M.D., *Refined Carbohydrate Foods and Disease* (London: Academic Press, 1975), p. 31.

11. Carlson Wade, *Miracle Protein* (West Nyack, New Jersey: Parker Publishing Company, 1975), p. 59.

12. Carl I. Flath, *The Miracle Nutrient* (New York: Bantam, 1976), p. 31.

13. See Note 12, p. 52.

14. Mohamed A. Antar, MBBCh., M.S., Margaret A. Ohlson,

Ph.D., and Robert E. Hodges, M.D., "Perspectives in Nutrition," *American Journal of Clinical Nutrition,* March 1964, Vol. 14, p. 174.

15. See Note 10, p. 341.

CHAPTER 9

1. Roy C. Darlington, Ph.D., "Laxatives," *Handbook of Non-Prescription Drugs,* 1973 Edition (Washington, D.C.: American Pharmaceutical Association), p. 63.
2. See Note 1.
3. Neil S. Painter, M.D., "Diverticular Disease of the Colon," *Geriatrics,* February 1976, pp. 90, 91.
4. See Note 3, p. 90.
5. Denis P. Burkitt, M.D., and C. W. Graham-Stewart, M.D., "Haemorrhoids—Postulated Pathogenesis and Proposed Prevention," *Postgraduate Medical Journal,* September 1975, p. 633.
6. J. C. Goligher, M.D., *Surgery of the Anus, Rectum, and Colon,* Second Edition (Springfield, Illinois: Charles C. Thomas, 1967), p. 114.
7. Michael D. Levitt, M.D., "Intestinal Gas," *Postgraduate Medicine,* Vol. 57, No. 1, January, 1975, p. 77.
8. Denis P. Burkitt, M.D., "Hemorrhoids, Varicose Veins, and Deep Vein Thrombosis: Epidemiologic Features and Suggested Causative Factors," *Canadian Journal of Surgery,* September 1975, p. 487.
9. Frank Greve and Mary Walton (Knight News Wire), "Elvis' Constipation Triggered 'Attack'," *Santa Ana Register,* August 28, 1977.

CHAPTER 10

1. Roy C. Darlington, Ph.D., "Laxatives," *Handbook of Non-Prescription Drugs,* 1973 Edition (Washington, D.C.: American Pharmaceutical Association), p. 64.
2. Alan L. Otten, "Better Health," *The Wall Street Journal,* February 24, 1977.
3. Marion C. Pruitt, M.D., *Hemorrhoids* (St. Louis: The C. V. Mosby Company, 1938), p. 62.
4. See Note 3.

5. Joseph Franklin Montague, M.D., *The Modern Treatment of Hemorrhoids* (Philadelphia: J. B. Lippincott Company, 1926), p. 119.

6. See Note 3.

7. See Note 3.

8. Stanley DuBrin, M.D., and James Keenan, *Acupuncture and Your Health* (Chatsworth, California: Books For Better Living, 1974), p. 84.

CHAPTER 11

1. Robert T. Turell, M.D., *Diseases of the Colon and Anorectum,* Volume II (Philadelphia: W. B. Saunders, 1969), p. 907.

2. J. C. Goligher, M.D., *Surgery of the Anus, Rectum, and Colon,* Second Edition (Springfield, Illinois: Charles C. Thomas, 1967), p. 118.

3. "Findings, Opinions, and Orders," *Federal Trade Commission Decisions,* Volume 70 (U.S. Government Printing Office: Washington), p. 1528.

4. See Note 3, p. 1539.

5. See Note 3, pp. 1634–35.

6. See Note 3, p. 1635.

7. See Note 3, p. 1639.

8. See Note 3, p. 1543.

9. See Note 3, pp. 1543–44.

10. See Note 3, pp. 1544–45.

11. See Note 3, p. 1557.

12. See Note 3, pp. 1644–45.

13. See Note 3, pp. 1524–1647.

14. "Findings, Opinions, and Orders," *Federal Trade Commission Decisions,* Volume 71 (U.S. Government Printing Office: Washington, 1970), pp. 822–68.

15. "Findings, Opinions, and Orders," *Federal Trade Commission Decisions,* Volume 76 (U.S. Government Printing Office: Washington), pp. 80–87.

16. "Findings, Opinions, and Orders," *Federal Trade Commission Decisions,* Volume 77 (U. S. Government Printing Office: Washington), pp. 728–30.

17. "Grove Laboratories, a division of Bristol-Myers, Petitioner versus Federal Trade Commission, Respondent," *Federal Re-*

porter, Volume 418, 2nd Series (U. S. Government Printing Office: Washington), pp. 489–98.

18. The Editors of Consumer Reports, *The Medicine Show* (New York: Pantheon Books, 1974), p. 106.

19. Thaddeus S. Grosicki, Ph.D. and K. Richard Knoll, Ph.D., "Hemorrhoidal Preparations," *Handbook of Non-Prescription Drugs,* 1973 Edition (Washington, D.C.: American Pharmaceutical Association), p. 151.

CHAPTER 12

1. Roy C. Darlington, Ph.D., "Laxatives," *Handbook of Non-Prescription Drugs,* 1973 Edition (Washington, D.C.: American Pharmaceutical Association), p. 63.

2. Louis A. Buie, Sr., M.D., *Practical Proctology,* Second Edition (Springfield, Illinois: Charles C. Thomas, 1960), pp. 219, 220.

3. The Editors of Consumer Reports, *The Medicine Show,* Revised Edition (New York: Pantheon Books, 1974), p. 99.

4. Marion C. Pruitt, M.D., *Hemorrhoids* (St. Louis: The C. V. Mosby Company, 1938), p. 61.

5. Joseph Franklin Montague, M.D., *The Modern Treatment of Hemorrhoids* (Philadelphia: J. B. Lippincott Company, 1926), p. 120.

6. See Note 5.
7. See Note 1, p. 62.
8. See Note 3, p. 101.
9. See Note 1, p. 62.
10. See Note 3, p. 94.
11. See Note 3, p. 94.
12. See Note 1.
13. See Note 1, p. 64.
14. See Note 1, p. 73.
15. See Note 1, p. 73.
16. See Note 1, p. 73.
17. See Note 1, p. 73.
18. See Note 1, pp. 64, 69.
19. See Note 1, p. 69.
20. See Note 1, p. 69.
21. See Note 1, p. 70.

22. See Note 1, p. 70.
23. See Note 1, p. 71.
24. See Note 1, p. 71.
25. See Note 1, p. 72.
26. See Note 1, p. 72.
27. See Note 1, p. 72.
28. See Note 1, p. 64.
29. See Note 3, p. 101.
30. See Note 3, p. 100.

CHAPTER 13

1. Roy C. Darlington, Ph.D., "Laxatives," *Handbook of Non-Prescription Drugs,* 1973 Edition (Washington, D.C.: American Pharmaceutical Association), p. 75.
2. See Note 1, p. 76.
3. The Editors of Consumer Reports, *The Medicine Show,* Revised Edition (New York: Pantheon Books, 1974), p. 100.
4. See Note 1.
5. See Note 1.
6. See Note 3.
7. See Note 1.
8. See Note 3.
9. See Note 1.

CHAPTER 14

1. Denis P. Burkitt, M.D., "Hemorrhoids, Varicose Veins, and Deep Vein Thrombosis: Epidemiologic Features and Suggested Causative Factors," *Canadian Journal of Surgery,* September 1975, p. 488.
2. Denis P. Burkitt, M.D., and C. W. Graham-Stewart, M.S., "Haemorrhoids: Postulated Pathogenesis and Proposed Prevention," *Postgraduate Medical Journal,* September, 1975, p. 635.
3. Joseph Franklin Montague, M.D., *The Modern Treatment of Hemorrhoids* (Philadelphia: J. B. Lippincott, 1926), p. 120.
4. John J. O'Connor, M.D. "Pediatric Proctology," *Diseases of the Colon and Rectum,* March 1975, p. 126.

5. Hamish Thomson, M.D., "Piles, Their Nature and Management," *The Lancet,* September 13, 1975, p. 494.

6. See Note 3, p. 126.

CHAPTER 16

1. E. Aubrey Cox, M.D., *Bottoms Up* (Durham, North Carolina: Moore Publishing Company, 1969), pp. 15, 16.

2. J. C. Goligher, M.D., *Surgery of the Anus, Rectum, and Colon,* Second Edition (Springfield, Illinois: Charles C. Thomas, 1967), p. 118.

3. J. P. Partridge, M.D., "Treatment of Haemorrhoids," *Nursing Times,* June 12, 1975, p. 928.

4. Joann S. Lublin, "Lighting the Way, Fiber Optics Research Spawns a Host of Uses in Medicine, Industry," *The Wall Street Journal,* November 30, 1976, p. 1.

CHAPTER 17

1. Martin I. Lewis, M.D., Teofilio De LaCruz, M.D., D. A. Gazzaniga, M.D., and Thomas L. Ball, M.D., "Cryosurgical Hemorrhoidectomy: Preliminary Report," *Diseases of the Colon and Rectum,* September–October 1969, p. 371.

2. Martin I. Lewis, M.D., "Cryosurgical Hemorrhoidectomy: A Follow-up Report," *Diseases of the Colon and Rectum,* March–April 1972, p. 128.

3. Martin I. Lewis, M.D., "Cryohemorrhoidectomy," *Diseases of the Colon and Rectum,* May–June 1973, p. 175.

4. H. D. Kaufman, M.D., "Cryotherapy for Piles," *British Medical Journal,* November 25, 1975, p. 463.

5. J. J. Bernhard, D.O., "Cryosurgical Hemorrhoidectomy: Pros and Cons," *Journal of the American Osteopathic Association,* November 1975, p. 344.

6. K. Lloyd Williams, M.D., "Cryodestruction of Haemorrhoids," *British Medical Journal,* March 17, 1973, p. 666.

7. Sanford Savin, M.D., "The Role of Cryosurgery in Management of Anorectal Disease: Preliminary Report on Results," *Diseases of the Colon and Rectum,* May–June 1975, p. 295.

8. Arthur A. Rand, M.D., "Symposium: Treatment of Hemor-

rhoids and Fissures," *Contemporary Surgery,* November 1973, p. 106.

9. William W. H. Rudd, M.D., "Symposium: Treatment of Hemorrhoids and Fissures," *Contemporary Surgery,* November 1973, p. 84.

10. John J. O'Connor, M.D., "Cryohemorrhoidectomy: Indications and Complications," *Diseases of the Colon and Rectum,* January–February 1976, p. 42.

11. See Note 2, p. 130.

12. Changyul Oh, M.D., "Treatment of Hemorrhoids and Applications of Cryotechnique," *Mt. Sinai Journal of Medicine,* March 1974, p. 194.

13. James Barron, M.D., "Ligation With Cryotherapy," *Diseases of the Colon and Rectum,* May–June 1973, p. 178.

14. Salvatore J. Detrano, M.D., "The Role of Cryosurgery in Management of Anorectal Diseases: Three Hundred and Fifty Cases," *Diseases of the Colon and Rectum,* May–June 1975, p. 285.

15. See Note 1, p. 373.

16. See Note 6, p. 667.

17. See Note 14, p. 284.

18. Stanley P. Wegryn, M.D., "Cryosurgery for Hemorrhoids," *Journal for the Medical Society of New Jersey,* December 1975, p. 1019.

19. Personal Communication, Sanford Savin, M.D., August 2, 1977.

20. Sanford Savin, M.D., "Hemorrhoidectomy—How I Do It: Results of 444 Cryorectal Surgical Operations," *Diseases of the Colon and Rectum,* April 1977, p. 189.

21. John J. O'Connor, M.D., "A Study of Cryosurgical Techniques," *Diseases of the Colon and Rectum,* May–June 1975, p. 298.

22. Bert Myers, M.D., and William Donovan, "Cryohemorrhoidectomy: An Experimental Study and Clinical Appraisal," *The American Surgeon,* December 1975, p. 799.

23. See Note 18.

24. See Note 5.

25. See Note 7, pp. 294–96.

26. Changyul Oh, M.D., and David A. Dreiling, M.D., "Cryo-

hemorrhoidectomy," *Mt. Sinai Journal of Medicine,* October 1974, p. 663.

27. See Note 14, p. 285.
28. See Note 22.
29. See Note 12.
30. See Note 12, p. 179.
31. Personal Communication, Sanford Savin, M.D., August 2, 1977.
32. See Note 7, p. 294.
33. Changyul Oh, M.D., "Cryohemorrhoidectomy Evaluated," *Diseases of the Colon and Rectum,* May–June 1975, p. 290.
34. See Note 13, p. 179.
35. See Note 26, p. 659.
36. See Note 12, p. 199.
37. See Note 18.
38. See Note 26, pp. 661–63.
39. See Note 13, p. 179.
40. See Note 14, p. 287.
41. See Note 33.
42. See Note 7, p. 296.
43. See Note 1, p. 374.
44. See Note 18.
45. See Note 2, pp. 130, 131
46. See Note 22, p. 803.
47. See Note 1, p. 374.
48. See Note 2, p. 131.
49. See Note 6, p. 667.
50. Salvatore J. Detrano, M.D., "Cryosurgical Hemorrhoidectomy," *Contemporary Surgery,* September, 1973.
51. See Note 7, p. 293.
52. See Note 12, p. 193.
53. See Note 7, p. 293.
54. See Note 21, p. 299.
55. See Note 26, p. 658.
56. See Note 5, p. 344.
57. See Note 6, p. 667.
58. See Note 12, p. 198.
59. See Note 4, p. 464.
60. See Note 18.

61. See Note 12, p. 198.
62. Personal Communication, Sanford Savin, M.D., July 18, 1977.
63. See Note 6, p. 667.
64. See Note 18.
65. See Note 12, p. 198.
66. See Note 62.
67. See Note 62.
68. Personal Communication, Changyul Oh, M.D., to Sanford Savin, M.D., July 18, 1977.
69. See Note 62.
70. See Note 7, p. 296.
71. See Note 2, p. 133.
72. See Note 26.
73. See Note 21, p. 299.
74. See Note 14, p. 286.
75. See Note 7, p. 295.
76. See Note 26, p. 660.
77. Leon Banov, Jr., M.D., "Backsides," *Archives of Surgery,* December, 1974.

ADDENDUM

1. Sanford Savin, M.D., "The Role of Cryosurgery in Management of Anorectal Disease: Preliminary Report on Results (Symposium)," *Diseases of the Colon and Rectum,* Vol. 18, 1975, p. 292.
2. Martin I. Lewis, M.D., Teofilio De LaCruz, M.D., D. A. Gazzaniga, M.D., et al., "Cryosurgical Hemorrhoidectomy: Preliminary Report," *Diseases of the Colon and Rectum,* Vol. 12, 1969, p. 371.
3. James Barron, M.D., "Diverse Methods of Managing Hemorrhoids: Ligation with Cryotherapy (Symposium)," *Diseases of the Colon and Rectum,* Vol. 16, 1973, p. 178.
4. Salvatore J. Detrano, M.D., "The Role of Cryosurgery in Management of Anorectal Disease: Three Hundred and Fifty Cases (Symposium)," *Diseases of the Colon and Rectum,* Vol. 18, 1975, p. 284.
5. Martin I. Lewis, M.D., "Cryosurgical Hemorrhoidectomy:

A Follow-up Report," *Diseases of the Colon and Rectum,* Vol. 15, 1972, p. 128.

6. John J. O'Connor, M.D. "The Role of Cryosurgery in Management of Anorectal Disease: A Study of Cryosurgical Techniques (Symposium)," *Diseases of the Colon and Rectum,* Vol. 18, 1975, p. 298.

7. John J. O'Connor, M.D., "Cryohemorrhoidectomy: Indications and Complications," *Diseases of the Colon and Rectum,* Vol. 19, 1976, p. 41.

8. Changyul Oh, M.D., "The Role of Cryosurgery in Management of Anorectal Disease: Cryohemorrhoidectomy Evaluated (Symposium)," *Diseases of the Colon and Rectum,* Vol. 18, 1975, p. 289.

9. Changyul Oh, M.D., "Treatment of Hemorrhoids and Application of Cryotechnique," *Mt. Sinai Journal of Medicine,* Vol. 42, 1975, p. 179.

10. W. H. Rudd, M.D., "Ligation of Hemorrhoids as an Office Procedure," *Canadian Medical Association Journal,* Vol. 108, 1973, p. 56.

11. K. L. Williams, I. U. Haq, and B. Elem, "Cryodestruction of Haemorrhoids," *British Medical Journal,* Vol. 1, 1973, p. 666.

Glossary

ABRASIONS—scrapings of the anal canal lining, evidenced by stools or slight bleeding during bowel movements.

ABSORPTION RATE—ability to absorb moisture.

ALIMENTARY CANAL—the passage of the body that food goes through, extending from the mouth to the anus.

ANAL CANAL—passageway leading from the rectum to the anus.

ANAL CUSHIONS—the three sponge-like pads forming a circle beneath the inner lining of the anal canal.

ANAL SKIN—term used to describe the modified anal skin, which forms the inner lining of the anal canal from the anus up to the pectinate line (approximately two-thirds the way up the anal canal).

ANAL VERGE—the circle of the anal opening at the anus.

ANEMIA—fatigued condition of the body, often due to a loss of blood.

ANESTHETIC—desensitizing ointment or drug given to provide patient comfort during a medical procedure.

ANORECTAL RING—boundary dividing the interior opening of the anal canal and the rectum.

ANOSCOPE—short, circular instrument used to examine the anal canal and rectum.

ANUS—exterior opening of the anal canal.

APPENDICITIS—inflammation of the appendix.

ARTERIOSCLEROSIS—a thickening and hardening of the walls of the arteries.

ARTERIOVENAL—describing arteries and veins which interconnect without the customary linking capillaries.

ARTERY—blood vessel carrying blood from the heart to all parts of the body.

BOWEL MOVEMENT—body wastes eliminated from the anus, also used to describe the passage of such wastes.

BOWELS—the lower alimentary tract, specifically the intestines.

BRAN—the outer skin of grains, indigestible in humans and having the propensity to absorb and retain moisture during its passage through the alimentary canal.

CAPILLARIES—tiny blood vessels connecting the arteries with the veins.

CARBOHYDRATES—foods derived from sugars and starches.

CATHARTICS—laxatives; sometimes used to describe strong laxatives.

CATHETERIZATION—insertion of slender tube into a body passage in order to draw off fluid (example: urine).

CAVITIES—sacs within the anal cushions which, when engorged with blood, effectively close the inner anal canal and are emptied by the forward-moving stools.

CELLULOSE—the chief substance composing the skin of plants.

CHOLESTEROL—substance produced by the body to lubricate the passage of blood in the circulatory system; also found in animal-protein foods. Excess levels of this substance may clog the blood vessels.

COLON—the large intestine, extending from the small intestine to the rectal pouch (rectum).

CONCEALED (OCCULT) BLOOD—blood appearing within the feces, not visible to the eye.

CONNECTIVE TISSUE—network of elastic tissue which helps anchor the anal cushions to the internal sphincter of the anal canal.

CONSTIPATION—condition in which the emptying of waste matter from the bowels is infrequent and difficult.

CONSTRICTION—a contraction or tightening of a body passage.

CONTRACTION—see "constriction."

CORONARY THROMBOSIS—formation of a clot in one of

the coronary arteries, resulting in the obstruction of the artery.

CRYOGENICS—a branch of physics that relates to the production and effects of very low temperatures.

CRYOHEMORRHOIDECTOMY—treatment of hemorrhoidal tissue with use of a freezing agent applied with a cryoprobe.

CRYOPROBE—instrument utilized to deliver the freezing effect.

CRYOSURGERY—see "cryohemorrhoidectomy."

CRYOTHERAPY—see "cryohemorrhoidectomy."

CUSHIONS—see "anal cushions."

DEEP VEIN THROMBOSIS—blood clot occurring in vein within the body.

DEFECATION—elimination of waste matter (feces) from the body.

DERMATOLOGY—branch of medicine dealing with the skin and its diseases.

DESCENDING COLON—the last third of the large intestine, leading downward to the rectum.

DESENSITIZING AGENT—anesthetic applied for the comfort of the patient.

DIABETES—disorder of the body characterized by excess of sugar in the blood and urine.

DIGESTIVE JUICES—juices secreted by the mouth to aid digestion.

DILATION—the act of making larger or wider, expanding.

DIRECT FREEZING—the freezing of hemorrhoidal tissue without the use of ligation.

DIVERTICULAR DISEASE—disorder of the colon, the formation of pouches or sacs opening out from the wall of the intestine.

ELASTIC TISSUE—see "connective tissue."

ENDOSPERM—the heart of the grain kernel, in wheat 83 percent of the bulk.

ENEMA—liquid or suppository, delivered into the rectum to encourage a bowel movement or as a cleansing agent.

ENGORGEMENT—the filling of the cavities of the anal canal cushions with blood, effectively closing the inner anal canal.

EPHEDRINE—chemical used to cause constriction of swollen or inflamed blood vessels.

EXCISION—removal by cutting.

EXTERNAL HEMORRHOIDS—fourth-degree hemorrhoids which permanently protrude from the anus and cannot be replaced within the anal canal; not to be confused with blood clots, a temporary condition, or skin tags.

EXTERNAL SPHINCTER—the voluntary muscle by which we consciously control the outer opening (anus) of the anal canal.

FALSE URGES—false sensations caused by prolapsed hemorrhoids after a bowel movement, which encourage the patient to remain on the toilet stool unnecessarily.

FECAL MATTER—waste matter, feces, stools, bowel movement.

FIBER—the indigestible food matter of grains, legumes, vegetables, and fruits which aids elimination by adding bulk to the feces.

FISSURE—a cleft or crack in the lining of the anal canal, often the source of anal pain and/or bleeding.

FISTULA—abnormal hollow passage from an abscess, cavity, or hollow organ to the skin or to another abscess, cavity, or organ.

FLATULENCE—see "flatus."

FLATUS—gas in the stomach or intestines, often resulting in the passage of excess gas from the anal canal.

GASTRIC JUICES—juices secreted in the stomach to aid digestion.

GERM—the embryo of the grain kernel, 2½ percent of the wheat kernel.

GUIAC PAPER TEST—a test for blood within the feces, accomplished by taking sample smears of the feces.

HEMICELLULOSES—portions of indigestible fiber which

have the ability to absorb large amounts of moisture.

HEMOCCULT TEST—see "guiac paper test."

HEMORRHAGE—bleeding.

HEMORRHOIDECTOMY—removal or elimination of hemorrhoidal tissue.

HEMORRHOIDS—*First Degree:* small bulges which do not prolapse. *Second Degree:* larger bulges which prolapse during a bowel movement but return of their own accord after the bowel movement. *Third Degree:* bulges which remain prolapsed at the conclusion of the bowel movement and require manual replacement. This type of prolapse may also occur while walking, during exercise, and with prolonged standing. *Fourth Degree:* hemorrhoids which due to their advanced size can no longer be replaced within the anus.

HIATUS HERNIA—protrusion of a part of the intestine through the abdominal muscles.

ICEBALL—formed by the application of the cryoprobe to body tissue.

ILEOCECAL SPHINCTER—muscular sphincter which permits the passage of waste material from the small intestine to pass into the large intestine (colon); primary function is to prevent the backflow of waste matter.

INGURGITATE—to pour into; the inflow of blood into the cavities of the anal cushions.

INTERNAL SPHINCTER—the involuntary muscle controlling the internal opening of the anal canal from the rectum.

INTESTINAL TRACT—lower part of the alimentary canal extending from the stomach to the anus.

LAXATIVES—medicine or substance taken to make the bowels loose and relieve constipation.

LEFT LATERAL POSITION—position of the patient lying on the left hip and shoulder, with the knees drawn up slightly.

LETHARGY—dull, sluggish state due to illness, fatigue, etc.

LIGATION—method of treating hemorrhoidal tissue by placing an elastic band around the base, thereby limiting the circulation of blood therein.

LIGNIN—portion of indigestible fiber, 9 percent of grain fibers.

LIQUEFACTION—process in which body tissue is reduced by being liquefied, the result of direct freezing method.

MASTICATION—the chewing of food matter within the mouth.

MODIFIED ANAL SKIN—see "anal skin."

MUCOSA—the lining of the inner third of the anal canal; also describes the lining of the rectum, a mucous membrane.

MUCOUS MEMBRANE—see "mucosa."

NATURAL RESOLUTION—the process in which the body naturally heals an inflammation without outside assistance (example: a blood clot).

OCCULT—concealed, not normally noticeable.

PECTINATE LINE—boundary dividing the outer two-thirds (anal skin) of the anal canal from the inner third (mucosa).

PERISTALSIS—the rhythmic, wavelike motion of the walls of the alimentary canal that move the contents forward.

PHENYLEPHRINE—chemical used to cause constriction of swollen or inflamed blood vessels.

PHYTIC ACID—substance occurring in grains and legumes which reduces the absorption of iron in the small intestines.

PILES—another term for hemorrhoids, frequently used in British medical terminology.

PORTAL PLETHORA—engorgement of veins leading to the liver from the rectal area.

PORTAL VEINS—veins leading to the liver from the rectal area.

POSTOPERATIVE—period following a medical procedure.

PROCTOLOGIST—physician specializing in disorders of the lower bowels.

PROCTOSCOPY—examination of the anal canal and rectum, utilizing a short telescopic instrument.

PROLAPSE—to protrude from the anal opening (anus).

PROTRUSIONS—portions of hemorrhoidal tissue in a prolapsed position.

RECTAL REFLEX—reflex of the body caused by the delivery of sufficient fecal matter into the rectum, resulting in an urge for a bowel movement.

RECTAL POUCH—the end of the large intestine at which fecal matter collects just prior to elimination.

RECTUM—see "rectal pouch."

REPLACEMENT—the replacing of prolapsed tissue within the anus.

RESIDUE—another word for indigestible food fiber.

ROLLER MILLS—machines used to separate and grind (refine) the components of grains.

SIGMOID COLON—that portion of the lower colon (large intestine) which makes an S-curve toward the center and rear of the abdomen and ends at the rectum.

SITZ BATHS—warm baths in three to four inches of water.

SKIN TAGS—tags of skin located at the margin of the anus, often the remnants of a blood clot or previous treatment for hemorrhoids.

SLOUGH—a mass of dead tissue which separates from the surrounding tissue; the act of shedding dead tissue.

SMALL INTESTINE—body organ which receives food matter from the stomach for further digestion, and then passes wastes on to the large intestine (colon).

SPHINCTERS—a ring-shaped muscle that surrounds a natural opening in the body, controlling such passage by expanding and contracting.

STOOL—waste matter expelled from the bowels; feces.

STOOL TEST—see "guiac paper test."

STRANGULATED HEMORRHOID—a prolapsed hemorrhoid which has remained in a prolapsed position so long that the external sphincter muscle has cut off the blood supply to the tissue, requiring immediate medical attention; not to be confused with a blood clot.

STRICTURE—a constriction of the anal canal, often resulting from continual inadequate dilation of the anal canal by poorly formed stools.

SUPPOSITORY—a small piece of medicated substance, intended to assist with a bowel movement, and introduced into the rectum where it is melted and diffused by the body temperature.

THROMBOSIS—coagulation of blood in some part of the circulatory system, forming a clot which obstructs circulation.

TRADITIONAL MEDICAL TREATMENT—excisional surgery, or the cutting out of hemorrhoidal tissue.

ULCERS—an abscess or wound on the skin or mucous membrane.

UNPROCESSED MILLER'S BRAN—bran fiber in its natural state.

URINARY RETENTION—inability to urinate.

VALVES—in the veins; backup valves which prevent the backward flow of blood.

VARICOSE VEIN—an abnormally and irregularly swollen or dilated vein.

VASCULAR—body tissue having numerous vessels for the passage of blood (example: the anal cushions).

VASOCONSTRICTOR—a drug causing constriction of the blood vessels.

VEINS—those blood vessels which return blood to the heart from all parts of the body.

VENAL—of the veins.

Index